Color Atlas
of Laparoscopic Surgery

# Color Atlas of Laparoscopic Surgery

Friedrich Götz, M.D.
Head, Division of Laparoscopic Surgery
Department of Surgery,
Grevenbroich Hospital
Teaching Hospital of the Technical
University (RWTH) Aachen
Grevenbroich, Germany

Arnold Pier, M.D.
Division of Laparoscopic Surgery
Department of Surgery,
Grevenbroich Hospital
Teaching Hospital of the Technical
University (RWTH) Aachen
Grevenbroich, Germany

Ekkehard Schippers, M.D., Ph.D.
Department of Surgery
Technical University (RWTH)
Aachen, Germany

Volker Schumpelick, M.D., Ph.D.
Professor and Chairman,
Department of Surgery
Technical University (RWTH)
Aachen, Germany

Foreword by Karl A. Zucker, M.D.

183 illustrations, most in color

1993
Georg Thieme Verlag
Stuttgart · New York

Thieme Medical Publishers, Inc.
New York

*Friedrich Götz, M.D.*
Head, Division of Laparoscopic Surgery
Department of Surgery
KKH Grevenbroich
Lehrkrankenhaus der RWTH
Von-Werth-Strasse 5
4048 Grevenbroich 1
Germany

*Arnold Pier, M.D., Dipl.-Ing.*
Division of Laparoscopic Surgery
Department of Surgery
KKH Grevenbroich
Lehrkrankenhaus der RWTH
Von-Werth-Strasse 5
4048 Grevenbroich 1
Germany

Photography: Michael Eikel, M.S.
Division of Laparoscopic Surgery
KKH Grevenbroich

Translated by Gerhard Sharon
4525 Henry Hudson Parkway
Riverdale, NY 10471
USA

*Ekkehard Schippers, M.D., Ph.D.*
Department of Surgery
Technical University
(RWTH) Aachen
Pauwelsstrasse
5100 Aachen
Germany

*Volker Schumpelick, M.D., Ph.D.*
Professor and Chairman, Department of Surgery
Technical University
(RWTH) Aachen
Pauwelsstrasse
5100 Aachen
Germany

This book is an authorized translation of the German edition published and copyrighted 1991 by Georg Thieme Verlag, Stuttgart, Germany.
Title of the German edition: Laparoskopische Chirurgie

*Library of Congress Cataloging-in-Publication Data*

[Laparoskopische Chirurgie]
Manual of laparoscopic surgery / Friedrich Goetz … [et al.].
   p.  cm.
   Includes bibliographical references and index.
   ISBN 3-13-791901-0 (G. Thieme Verlag). --
ISBN 0-86577-470-6
(Thieme Medical Publishers)
   1. Abdomen--Endoscopic surgery. 2. Gallblad-
der--Endoscopic surgery. 3. Appendix--Endoscop-
ic surgery. 4. Laparoscopy.
I. Götz, Friedrich.
   [DNLM: 1. Peritoneoscopy. 2. Surgery, Opera-
tive--methods. WI 575 L2995]
RD540.M   1992
617.5'5059--dc20
DNLM/DLC
for Library of Congress          92−49502
                              CIP



© 1993 Georg Thieme Verlag,
Rüdigerstrasse 14, 7000 Stuttgart 30, Germany
Thieme Medical Publishers, Inc., 381 Park Avenue
South, New York, N.Y. 10016
Typesetting and Printing by Druckhaus Götz GmbH,
D-7140 Ludwigsburg;
Typesetting on Linotype System 5 (202)
Printed in Germany

ISBN 3-13-791901-0 (GTV, Stuttgart)
ISBN 0-86577-470-6 (TMP, New York)     1 2 3 4 5 6

# Foreword

The impetus for this exceptional textbook "Color Atlas of Laparoscopic Surgery" was without a doubt the authors' enthusiasm and pioneering role in the development of laparoscopic cholecystectomy. Never before in the history of modern medicine has the introduction of a single operative procedure had such a profound effect on the practice of clinical surgery. Dr. Götz and his coauthors have contributed enormously to the field of laparoscopic surgery and this is clearly reflected in the contents of this atlas. The authors have written an extremely lucid and informative summary of the basic operative steps in performing a laparoscopic procedure, as well as an informative description of the techniques of laparoscopic cholecystectomy, intraoperative cholangiography, appendectomy, and adhesiolysis.

The impact of therapeutic laparoscopy extends far beyond its application for gallbladder surgery. With amazing swiftness surgeons have taken those skills learned by performing laparoscopic cholecystectomy and used them to apply this technology in the management of common bile duct stones, acute appendicitis, gastroesophageal reflux, and peptic ulcer disease, as well as in the treatment of various benign and malignant disorders of the colon. Thus far, the benefits of diminished postoperative pain, shorter hospital stays, and faster recovery have been realized in all of these laparoscopic procedures. It is conceivable, therefore, that within a few years operative procedures utilizing laparoscopic technology may represent the majority of the gastrointestinal surgeon's clinical practice. The impact of such a dramatic change in the practice of surgery is eagerly anticipated by some but rather frightening to others. Clearly not every surgeon will be as adept and skillful at operating through tiny holes while looking at a two-dimensional video screen as the authors of this textbook. How will such individuals face the consequences of such changes? Another as yet unanswered question is: how will surgeons learn these tedious and complicated laparoscopic techniques once they have completed their surgical training? Another question is implied by the chapter on instrumentation: will the costs of this sophisticated technology and the increasing popularity of disposable laparoscopic equipment negate the expected benefits of reduced health care expenses?

Clearly such answers are beyond the scope of this or any other textbook of surgery. The more immediate challenge for those individuals who are currently performing laparoscopy or planning to learn such skills in the near future is to acquire as much information as possible regarding the technical aspects and potential complications associated with this type of surgery. This text would clearly help such individuals to achieve these goals.

*Karl A. Zucker, M.D., FACS*

*Professor of Surgery*
*University of New Mexico School of Medicine*

# Preface

Innovations in a specialty that is rich in tradition almost invariably pass through phases of initial rejection, critical evaluation, cautious, then often enthusiastic, approval and finally, consolidation of proven findings. Each phase has its own time, its own self-appointed protagonist, and its own rationale. Laparoscopic surgery is in the midst of this development. Controlled findings are lacking, one camp voices skepticism and the other enthusiastic approval, and it is too early to draw even preliminary conclusions. Yet the evolution of a new surgical discipline is beginning to become apparent even now.

Given this state of affairs, we thought it desirable to give a clean description and a visual demonstration of the practical knowledge we have gained thus far. The indications and techniques we use, our experience, and the problems we have encountered are offered in review to help others in their efforts to start with the basic techniques and proven methods of laparoscopic surgery. We do not aim to render our total experience in laparoscopic surgery in exhaustive detail nor to give a complete analysis of the data in the literature. Many new laparoscopic surgical procedures have been described in the last 2 years; many new, mostly disposable, instruments have been developed. We cannot include them all, as we have chosen to focus on the basics of laparoscopic surgery. The presentation is geared toward practical issues, designed to facilitate the beginner's first steps and to allow those more advanced in the art to compare different methods.

We would like to express our heartfelt thanks to Felicien Steichen, M.D., for reviewing the English translation and making many invaluable suggestions.

We are also indebted to Dr. Günther Hauff, Georg Thieme Verlag, for publishing this book and, above all, to his associates for their excellent cooperation and the swift realization of this project.

Aachen, October 1992    V. Schumpelick

# Table of Contents

# Introduction

The goal of modern techniques in surgery is to achieve optimal therapeutic results while tissue integrity and organ function are minimally disturbed by the operative treatment. "Nil nocere suprema lex" is the motto; physiologically functional restoration through anatomically appropriate repairs is the maxim. These aims have led surgeons away from radical excisions for malignancy if statistically valid reasons at comparable levels of tumor staging favor tissue saving or "economical" resections. The tendency of preserving form and function—or parts thereof—is enhanced by the availability and continuous development of immediate or delayed early reconstructive procedures, with biological tissues or prosthetic devices, in an ever-increasing array of patients with diseases of various etiologies.

Laparoscopy, allowing extensive visual and procedural exposure of the abdominal cavity through a reduced, "atraumatic" anatomical access, fits harmoniously within this overall approach to the diagnosis and surgical treatment of various intra-abdominal conditions. The reserved attitude and nescient rejection of yesterday have given way to feverish efforts at keeping pace with ever accelerating developments. Overnight laparoscopy has become "socially" acceptable, as it were. Equipped with modern instrumentation, a visual field that is projected onto a TV monitor (so typical of our era), and supported by computerized technology, today's laparoscopy meets the requirements of "high-tech" surgery. Rarely has surgery been overtaken by so tempestuous a development as the massive conversion to laparoscopic cholecystectomy during the past few years.

The reasons for this are varied: the desire for innovative improvements in a tradition-bound discipline, the competition with alternative methods of gallstone therapy, the acceptance and preference by patients, and the intensifying struggle for a share of health care expenditures. Abdominal surgery is only now catching up with gynecology, urology, neurosurgery, traumatology, and orthopedics which have added less invasive, endoscopic operative procedures to their array of therapeutic modalities a long time ago. Surgeons are learning to replace the formulation of diagnosis and therapy based on palpation of the affected organ by decisions obtained through magnified visualization and a tactile sense transmitted through interposed instruments.

Video-guided or -assisted surgery will not eliminate the need for hand–eye coordination but complement and enhance it under well-defined circumstances and spare the patient from the discomfort and consequences of a traditional incision. Technical perfection and a strict definition of indications remain foremost surgical precepts; the need to avoid complications and unnecessary risks is self-evident. Laparoscopic surgery is not "minor surgery" but "major surgery through a small incision," broadened by the spatial impression of two dimensions and the mental projection of a third one provided by the magnified image transmitted from the optical systems to the video screen with a great accuracy of detail. Research in progress will soon provide the operating team with a true, three-dimensional picture.

These advantages are gained at a considerable cost in personnel and material. Conventionally trained surgical personnel need to be persuaded, and then administrators will complain that the new types of operations exceed budgetary limitations because of the cost of the basic equipment and the use of disposable instruments. Abdominal surgery, which has until now managed to operate with reusable, traditional instruments going back to Kocher, Roux, Péan, Cooper, Langenbeck, Dupuytren, Mikulicz, Halsted, and Mayo, among many others, is now compelled to work with expensive, disposable products of different suppliers. It is to be hoped that this will not offset the otherwise cost-reducing effect of the new methods in shortening the duration of hospitalization.

Endoscopically guided intracavitary and endoluminal surgical procedures pose a timely challenge to traditional surgical techniques. But this challenge does not endanger accepted principles of surgical thought and action nor does it represent a different or radically diminished expression of surgical therapy. It is merely a new bud in the perenially growing garden of surgical flowers.

# The History of Laparoscopy

Finds from antiquity in Greece and Italy attest to mankind's early interest in examining the cavities of the human body. Tubelike instruments, so-called specula, were found in the ruins of Pompeii which were used for the study of the vagina and inspection of the cervix, for examination of the rectum, and for an inside view of the nose and ear.

Subsequently, Abulkasim of Cordoba (980−1037) and, later on, Giulio Cesare Aranzi (1530−1589) attempted to illuminate deeper body cavities through the reflection of natural light or by use of the camera obscura. The true origins of contemporary laparoscopy are traceable to the development of the cystoscope in the 19th century. Introduction of the light conductor by Bozzini (1805) (Fig. **1**) as modified by the Frenchman Desormeaux (1853) led to the first practical cystoscope, which still had to be used without a system of lenses, however.

The decisive step in the development of the endoscope was taken by Nitze (1879), who combined a cystoscope with the incandescent lamp just invented by Edison (Fig. **2**). Concurrently, systematic exploration of the body cavities was initiated at the beginning of the 20th century. While von Ott (1909) in St. Petersburg carried out his first endoscopic inspection of the abdominal cavity by way of a minilaparotomy, Kelling, a disciple of Mikulicz, used for the first time a Nitze−Leiter cystoscope that he had developed to examine the organs of the abdominal cavity. He performed the first full-fledged laparoscopy.

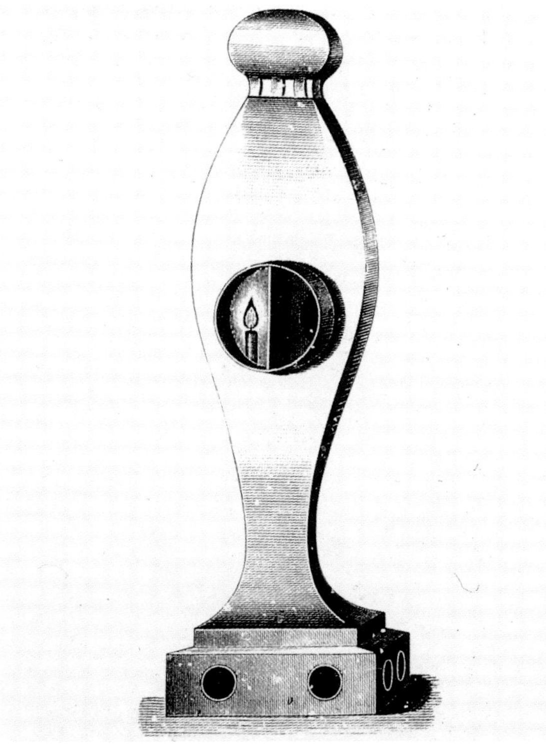

Fig. **1** "Light conductor" by Bozzini (1805). With the aid of a concave mirror the light from a wax candle was projected into the cavity to be investigated.

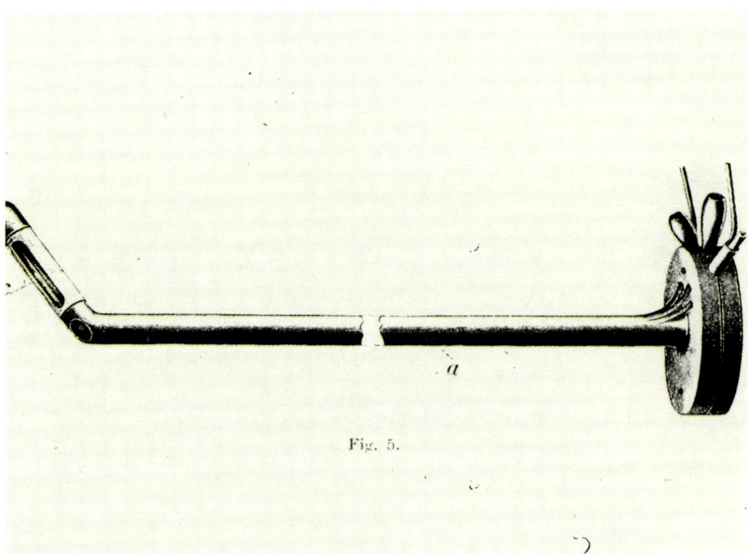

Fig. **2**  Cystoscope by Nitze (1879). The combination of the endoscope with the incandescent lamp invented by Edison made possible for the first time the illumination of hollow organs by shifting the light source to the interior of the body.

In addition, Kelling demonstrated in animal experiments that induction of a pneumoperitoneum was essential to carry out this examination, which he at that time called celioscopy.

Kelling's method attracted little attention at first but was taken up again by the Swede Jakobaeus (1910), who developed Kelling's ideas further, improved the instrumentation, and presented this new technique as laparoscopy. His personal experience with this new method was described in a monograph "Laparoscopy" (1912), which aroused considerable interest. One year later, reports were published from all over the world, providing evidence of the widespread use of the method. Additional developments centered on improvement of the instrumentation, such as the design of the trocar endoscope by Nordentoft (1912), the first needle for the induction of a pneumoperitoneum by Korbsch (1921), the invention of the insufflator by Goetze (1921), and the widening of the viewing angle through the laparoscope by Unverricht (1923). These advances in the instrumentation paved the way for even wider use of the method.

Laparoscopy attracted increasing clinical interest, mostly among internists at first, in the 1920s. Foremost in Germany is the hepatologist Kalk, who carried out a standardization of laparoscopy based on his considerable personal experience and who succeeded in establishing it as a routine procedure in internal medicine.

The first descriptions of operations performed under laparoscopic vision came from Fervers (1933). The next year, Stolze demonstrated for the first time the role of laparoscopy in a variety of surgical applications. In gynecology, Palmer in France, Decker in the United States of America, and Frangenheim and Semm in Germany made vital contributions to the establishment and perfection of laparoscopy, first as a diagnostic and later as a therapeutic procedure.

Although it continued to have individual advocates (Lindenschmidt 1963), laparoscopy soon fell into oblivion in surgery of the alimentary tract. Though optical developments (Hopkins 1976), employment of the glass fiber technique (Hirschowitz 1958), electronic control of the pneumoperitoneum (Semm 1980), the possibility of endocoagulation, and the use of special techniques such as endosuture and the Roeder loop (Semm 1978) broadened the range of gynecological laparoscopic operations, surgeons took little notice of these innovations. It was hardly surprising, therefore, that it was a gynecologist, Semm, who performed the first laparoscopic appendectomy in 1982.

Gynecologists thus deserve the credit for pioneering the newer developments during this transitional period. To orthodox surgeons, "buttonhole surgery" seemed less than reliable, too spectacular, not serious enough, and in a sense "unsurgical."

Not until the extension of laparoscopic techniques to the removal of the gallbladder by Mouret (1987), followed by the reports of Dubois et al. (1989), Perissat et al. (1990), Reddick and Olsen (1989), and Cuschieri (1990) did surgeons reenter the scene. Within a few months, laparoscopy awakened from its surgical dormancy and became the center of intense activity.

## Development of Operative Laparoscopy

| | |
|---|---|
| Bozzini 1805 | Light conductor |
| Desormeaux 1853 | Rectoscope and cystoscope |
| Nitze 1879 | Cystoscope with light source |
| Kelling 1901 | Celioscopy |
| Jakobaeus 1910 | First laparoscopy with pneumoperitoneum |
| Fervers 1933 | First laparoscopic adhesiolysis |
| Kalk 1962 | Standardization of diagnostic laparoscopy |
| Semm 1980 | Controlled pneumoperitoneum |
| Semm 1982 | First laparoscopic appendectomy |
| Mouret 1987 | First laparoscopic cholecystectomy |
| Götz 1988 | Standardization of laparoscopic appendectomy |
| Dubois<br>Perissat<br>Reddick<br>Götz } 1989 | Standardization of laparoscopic cholecystectomy |

# Education, Technical Preparation, and Material Conditions

## Surgeon and Assistant

Laparoscopic operations are full-blown surgical interventions, though they are performed under conditions beyond the range of a conventional operation. They are neither so-called minioperations, imposing reduced demands on the surgeon, nor do they represent low-risk minor surgical intervention. Special requirements have to be met for procedures of this type.

## Training and Experience in Abdominal Surgery

Mastery of the general and special basic rules of abdominal surgery is indispensable for every laparoscopic surgeon. This means that the surgeon and his or her first assistant must have the experience that enables them to continue the operation with the abdomen open, if necessary, at every stage of the laparoscopic procedure and to control any complications that may develop (injury of organs, hemorrhage, etc.).

## Training in Endoscopic Techniques and Visual Projection of Spatial Dimensions

The increased use of sophisticated technology, the unaccustomed approach, and the limited, two-dimensional image place added demands on the dexterity and spatial imagination of both the surgeon and the assistant. For this reason, knowledge and experience in endoscopic diagnosis and treatment are essential. Familiarity of an endoscopically knowledgeable surgeon with the two-dimensional picture permits rapid three-dimensional orientation in laparoscopy as well.

## Hands-on Training in Basic Steps

Even though the techniques of dissection and suture in laparoscopic operations do not differ fundamentally from those done through the open abdomen, their execution requires manual dexterity and constant practice. These are necessary because of the restricted range of action of the instruments that are advanced through the narrow circular pivot represented by the opening in the abdominal wall.

## Familiarity with the Instruments

Like all surgical techniques, reliable performance depends on exact knowledge of the instruments and their uses. Both the surgeon and the assistants must be able to handle their instruments blindly. Since not all the instruments can be seen at the same time, handling them individually in the absence of overall direct visual control takes practice.

## Eye (Camera and Monitor) and Hand Coordination

Another basic requirement for the trouble-free performance of laparoscopic operations is the coordinated manipulation of the camera, which represents the eyes of everyone taking part in

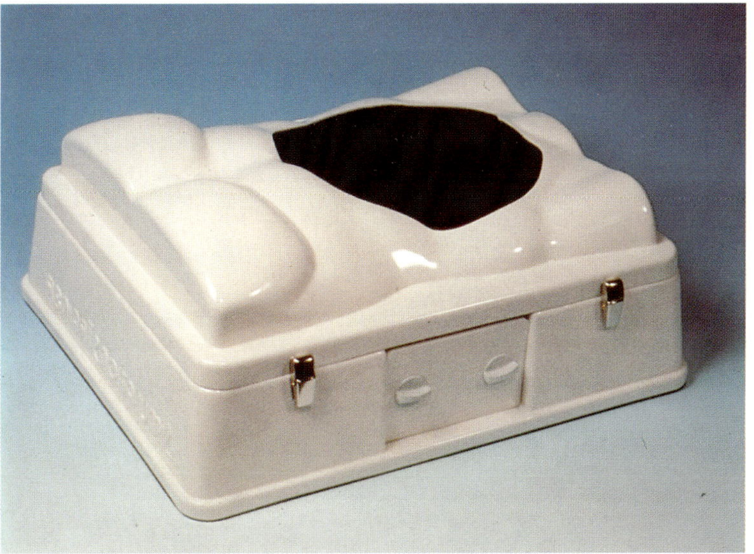

Fig. **3**  Simulation trainer for instruction in laparoscopic techniques including the induction of a pneumoperitoneum on a model and exercises on natural surgical specimens.

the operation. If the surgeon himself does not maneuver it, the assistant holding and directing the camera must know the exact sequence of the individual steps. Additionally, the assistant has to care for the smooth flow and progress of the procedure, particularly during a change of instruments, by securing and holding the trocar sheaths in the selected positions in the abdominal wall.

### Training with a Simulation Model

Step-by-step training on a model is strongly advised for every surgeon working in laparoscopy. At the beginning, systematic practice with a simulation trainer (Fig. **3**) is recommended in addition to the study of appropriate teaching films. This gives the assistant as well as the surgeon the opportunity to coordinate their respective participation in a three-dimensional space, seen in only two dimensions on the monitor. The basic techniques of laparoscopic surgery should be repeated with this device any number of times and thus learned, initially under direct vision and later with the aid of a video camera.

### Education by Apprenticeship

The next step is assistance in the performance of laparoscopic operations by an experienced surgeon. This provides an opportunity for carrying out individual steps, such as insertion of the Verres needle or of the trocars, under expert supervision. Independent performance of diagnostic laparoscopies should precede the operative intervention. Increased use of diagnostic laparoscopy for the evaluation of obscure abdominal complaints and in surgical oncology, within the context of tumor staging, for example, is an excellent means of perfecting the individual's laparoscopic technique.

## Nursing Staff

The rapid development ot laparoscopic surgery represents a challenge also for the operating room personnel. They should familiarize themselves, to the same extent as the surgeon, with the technical characteristics of the new equipment, the special instrumentation, and the operative steps. This task is made easier by the fact that the staff has the opportunity to follow every step of the operation on the video screen to the same extent as the surgeon (Fig. **4**).

This serves to enhance the participants' motivation and can well offset initial difficulties encountered by the nurses in learning to master the elaborate technical equipment. Nevertheless, the following conditions have to be met.

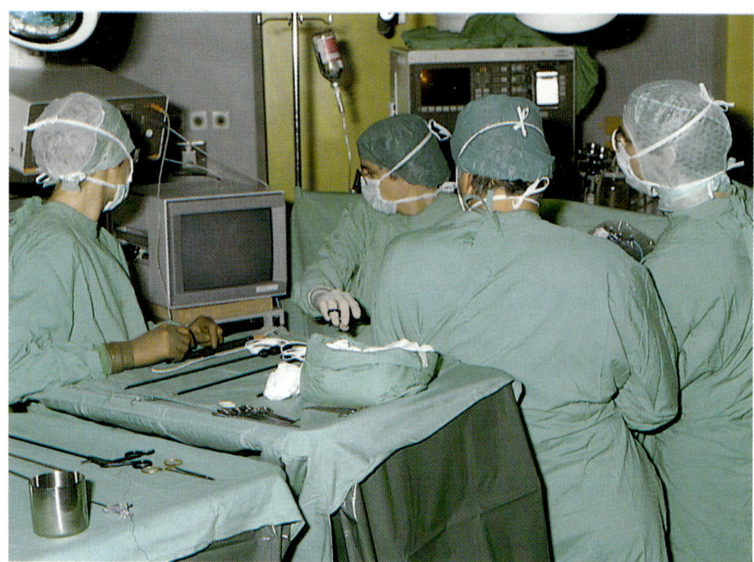

Fig. **4**  Reproduction of the intraoperative status on the TV monitor permits the surgical personnel to follow exactly the individual steps of the operation.

## Technical Assistance

Even more than for conventional laparotomy, the frequent adjustments of the settings on the insufflator, the light source, and the irrigation−suction equipment require the permanent presence of a technically proficient surgical nurse in the operating room.

## Maintenance of Equipment

The necessary cleaning and maintenance of the instrumentation, some of which is highly sensitive and fragile, require care and expertise which are generally lacking in a central supply and sterilization facility. Ideally, therefore, the operating room staff itself should be responsible for the care of the instruments. The use of disposable instruments solves this problem only partially, apart from being an important cost factor.

## Operative Assistance

All in all, the requirements to be met by the personnel in the performance of laparoscopic operations conform to the basic rules of abdominal surgery. In addition, special expertise and aptitudes are required which can rapidly become routine for everyone involved after appropriate training and regular participation in laparoscopic operations. Even more so than in laparotomy, coordinated team work is a certain condition for the successful performance of laparoscopic procedures.

## Basic Equipment and Instrumentation

The increasingly interventional nature of laparoscopic procedures has had a major impact on the development of the instruments in the past few years. It was preceded by the introduction of miniaturized video cameras, perfection of the electronically controlled $CO_2$ insufflator, and improvement of the lighting and optical systems. By now, the instruments are supplied by a growing number of manufacturers. For the technical design of individual instruments and their different features, reference may be made to detailed monographs. In what follows, we shall confine ourselves to a listing of the generic devices and basic instruments needed for day-to-day laparoscopic surgery.

## Insufflation Apparatus

Carbon dioxide is the gas most widely used in operative laparoscopy. Its advantages are good elimination via the lungs and low inflammability. Compared with air and laughing gas embolisation, emboli due to inadvertent $CO_2$ injection into a blood vessel can be controlled more easily. The maintenance of a constant pneumo-peritoneum at 12–15 mmHg is an essential condition for any interventional laparoscopy. However, the introduction of multiple trocars, in common with the frequent change of instruments, inevitably entails a loss of gas. In addition, every use of the suction apparatus is associated with a considerable decrease in intra-abdominal pressure because of the simultaneous aspiration of gas. The new generation of insufflators with high flow rates ranging up to 8 l/min and an electronically controlled, automatic switch for the loss of pressure does provides a high degree of assurance that the pneumoperitoneum will be maintained.

## Suction and Irrigation Apparatus

Suction and irrigation systems are essential components in laparoscopic surgery. The suction and irrigation devices available at present do permit their operation with one hand but could still be improved. In particular, better technical solutions are needed to deal with the substantial loss of gas, the aspiration of bits of tissue, and the frequent clogging of the aspirators with clots.

## Light Source, Optical System, and Video Unit

The use of halogen lamps with an output ranging up to 450 W ensures maximal illumination of the abdominal cavity. In conjunction with the high-resolution video-1-chip camera, a daylight-like picture is thus produced on the monitor (Fig. 5). An optimal image area is provided by a 10 mm, forward-viewing lens system. However, in some situations, a 30° viewing endoscope which can simply be rotated to change the angle of view proves advantageous.

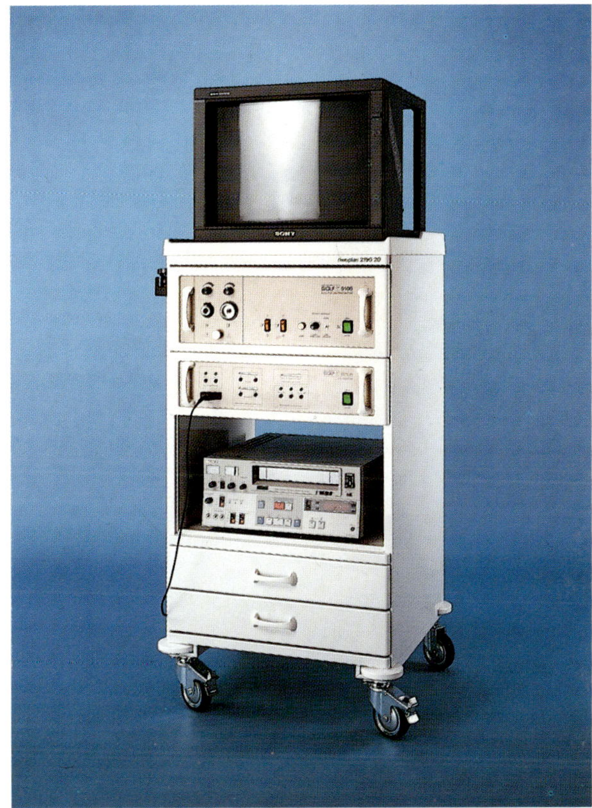

Fig. **5**  Mobile video unit with TV monitor, light source, camera, and video recorder. The $CO_2$ insufflator may also be carried within this unit.

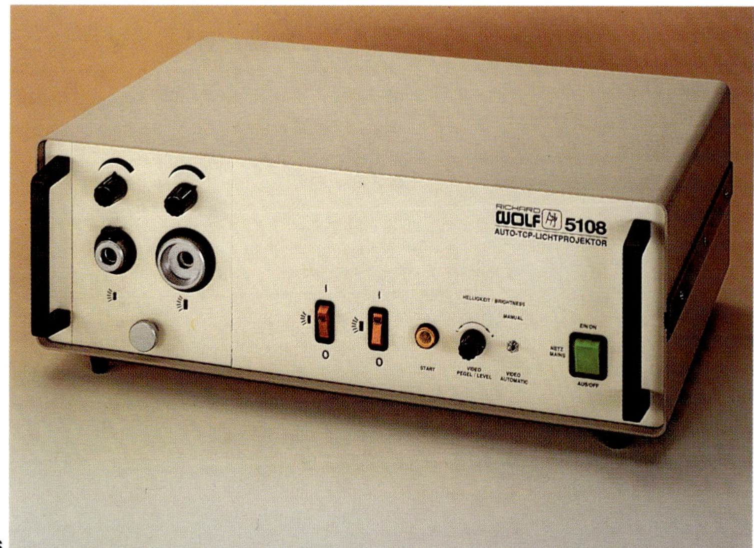
6

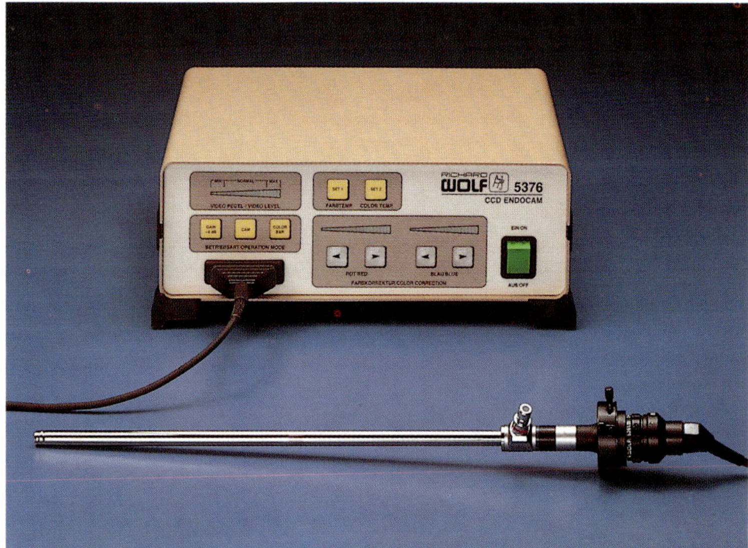
7

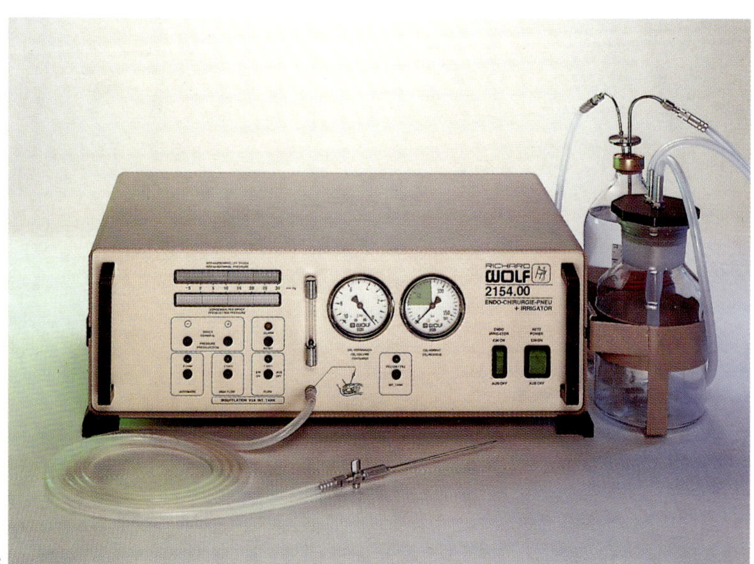
8

**Systemized Basic Equipment**
(Figs. **5–8**)

Video unit (Fig. **5**):
1  video monitor
1  video recorder: VHS, S-VHS, or
   U-Matic (optional)
1  video carriage (optional)
1  video printer (optional)

1  cold light source with halogen
   vapor arc lamp, 250–450 W
   (Fig. **6**)
1  fiberoptic light cable

1  miniature video camera (zoom
   optional)
   (Fig. **7**)
1  lens, 10 mm, 0° viewing
1  lens, 7 mm, 0° viewing
1  lens preheater

1  $CO_2$ insufflator (Fig. **8**)
   (pressure preselector, high-flow
   switch)
1  $CO_2$ bottle
1  set of tubes with Luer coupling
1  Verres needle
1  suction and irrigation apparatus
   including collecting bottle and
   tubing (Fig. **8**)
1  bipolar high-frequency electrocautery unit including con-
   necting cable
1  monopolar electrocautery unit
1  foot switch

## Instrumentation for Laparoscopic Appendectomy

(Fig. **9 a—c**)

1 trocar sheath, 11 mm, including trocar with trumpet valve (conical tip; Fig. **9 b**)
1 trocar sheath, 11 mm, including trocar with flap valve (triangular tip)
1 trocar sheath, 5 mm, including trocar with ball valve (triangular tip; Fig. **9 c**)
1 appendix extractor, 10 mm
1 grasping forceps, heavy
1 grasping forceps, atraumatic, 5 mm
1 bipolar grasping forceps
1 pair of scissors, 5 mm, straight
1 palpation rod, 5 mm, graduated
1 applicator, 5 mm
1 suction/irrigation tube, 5 mm

Optional:
1 pair of hooked scissors
1 dilator and guiding sheath, 10—15 mm
1 guide rod, 10 mm
1 trocar sheath, 15 mm outlet

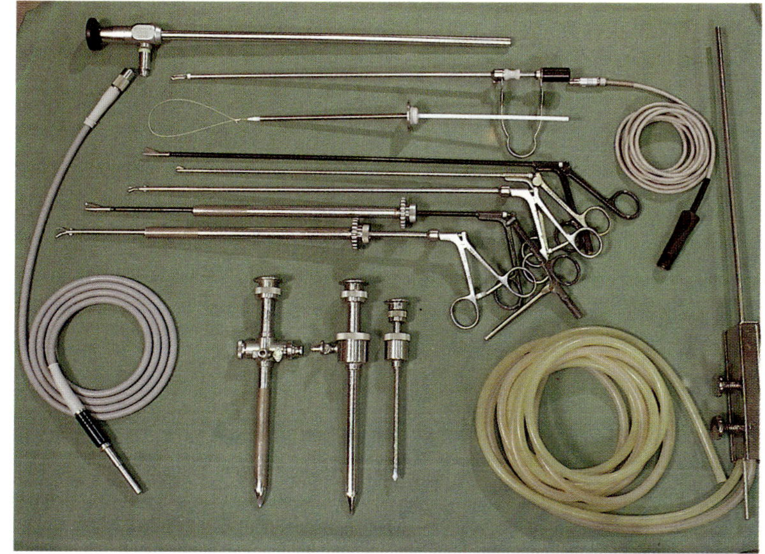

9a

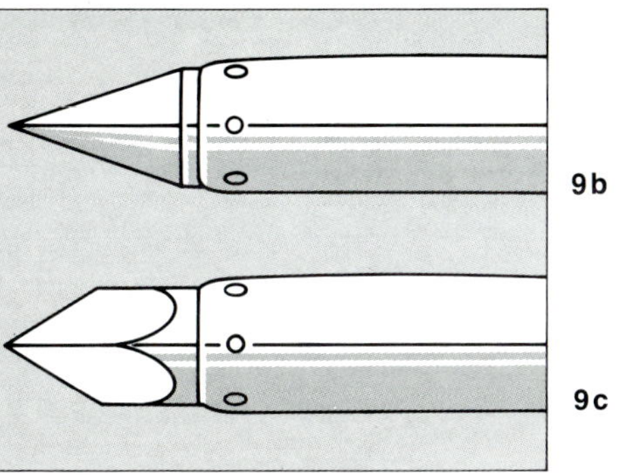

9b

9c

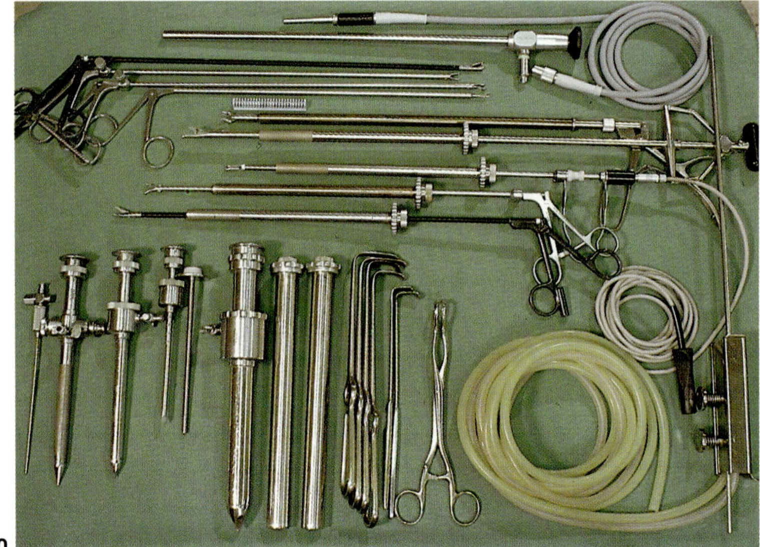

10

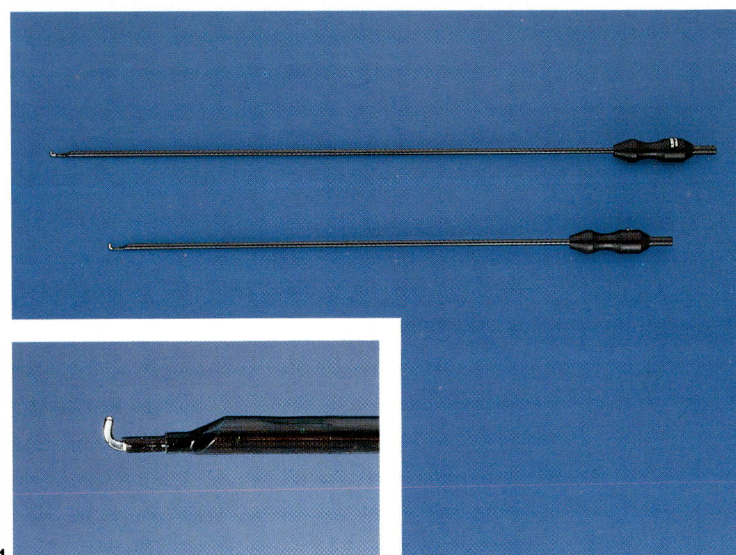

11

## Instrumentation for Laparoscopic Cholecystectomy
(Figs. **10, 11**)

1 trocar sheath, 11 mm, including trocar with trumpet valve (conical tip)
1 trocar sheath, 11 mm, including trocar with flap valve (triangular tip)
2 trocar sheaths, 5 mm, including trocar with flap valve (triangular tip)
2 instrumentation sheaths, 10 mm
1 palpation rod, graduated, 5 mm
1 pair of scissors, 5 mm, straight
1 clip applicator, including clips, possibly with guide sheath, 10 mm
1 grasping forceps, sharp
1 grasping forceps, atraumatic, 5 mm
1 suction/irrigation tube
1 grasping forceps, atraumatic, for gauze dissector
1 dissecting forceps, curved

Optional:
1 hooked electrode (Fig. **11**)
1 dilator and guiding sheath, 10 to 15/20 mm
1 guide rod, 10 mm
1 trocar sheath, 15 mm outlet

Supplementary instrumentation for cholangiography:
1 pair of dissecting microscissors, 5 mm
1 puncture needle, 5 mm
1 balloon catheter, 4−5 Fr

## Instrumentation for Laparoscopic Adhesiolysis
(Fig. **12**)

1 trocar sheath, 11 mm, including trocar with trumpet valve (conical tip)
2 trocar sheaths, 5 mm, including trocar with ball valve (triangular tip)
1 palpation rod, graduated, 5 mm
1 pair of scissors, 5 mm, straight
1 bipolar grasping forceps, 5 mm
1 loop applicator, 5 mm
1 suction/irrigation tube, 5 mm
1 grasping forceps, atraumatic
1 grasping forceps, heavy

Instrumentation for endosuture:
1 needle holder, 5 mm
1 needle holder, 10 mm, with converter

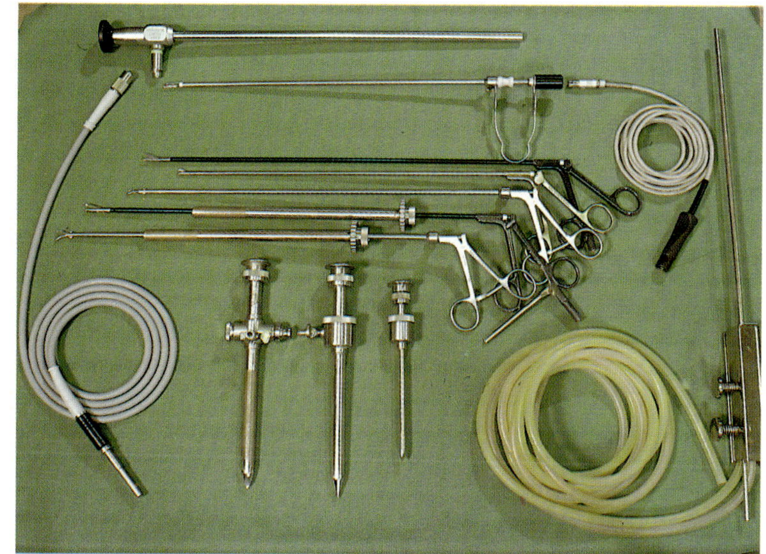

**12**

## Supplementary Instrumentation

As a general rule, the need for a changeover to laparotomy should be borne in mind in every laparoscopic operation. The instruments required for this purpose should be available without delay. An emergency kit for immediate laparotomy in particular should be at hand in case of uncontrollable intra-abdominal bleeding. The surgical instruments for the laparoscopy per se are limited to what is required for incision and closure of fascia and skin. For the extraction of the gallbladder, a gallbladder-grasping forceps, two short hooks, and variously curved forceps for stone extraction may be needed.

# Patient Preparation

## Information for the Patient

Fully informing the patient is the first step in patient preparation. The dialogue with the patient should include the details of a conventional operation. Besides describing the proposed procedure in general, with special reference to the organ involved and possible complications, the patient's attention should be drawn specifically to the unique features of the laparoscopic procedure. It is important to emphasize the initially diagnostic nature of laparoscopy. Also to be stressed is the fact that even if the preoperative diagnosis is confirmed, the final decision for or against a laparoscopic operation is only made intraoperatively. While leaving the patient with some uncertainty preoperatively, he or she should be aware of the advantages of a confirmed diagnosis and the reduced stress associated with diagnostic laparoscopy only. The potential need for a laparotomy should also be made emphatically clear. This should be explained to the patient in such a way that he or she will not interpret a changeover to laparotomy as a failure of the method or the surgeon, but rather as the optimal choice of procedure for his or her individual condition. This clear preoperative explanation will facilitate intraoperative decision-making. It is helpful in the postoperative guidance of the patient to mention preoperatively that the usually rapid return of subjective well-being cannot be considered a marker for internal wound healing.

## Preoperative Measures

### Preparation for Operation

Since the need for laparotomy may arise, the patient has to be prepared accordingly. This includes evaluation of the cardiorespiratory status, risks of general anesthesia, bowel preparation, hair removal, and washing of the abdominal wall. The umbilical fossa has to be cleaned with special care because the laparoscopic trocar is generally inserted paraumbilically. Disinfection during the evening before the operation by application of a povidone-iodine−impregnated swab to the umbilical fossa is helpful.

### Nasogastric Tube, Urinary Bladder Drainage

After intubation, a nasogastric tube is introduced routinely for decompression of the stomach. A distended stomach is at risk of being punctured by the Verres needle, and it obstructs the view in the upper abdomen. Another recommended safety measure is emptying of the bladder. Inadvertent puncture of the bladder and obstruction of view during exploration of the pelvis are thus prevented. Both the nasogastric tube and the bladder catheter are removed immediately after the operation.

## Positioning

For induction of the pneumoperitoneum, the patient is first placed in neutral dorsal decubitus before the procedure-specific adjustment of the operating table is carried out. Upper abdominal operations are facilitated by a reverse Trendelenburg position (10°−20°); conversely, a Trendelenburg position of 10°−20° is useful for the inspection and manipulation of the organs in the lower abdomen. Exposure of the left and right halves of the body is accomplished by a 10°−20° inclination of the table toward the side opposite the intended site of inspection. An intraoperative change in the patient's position requires good fixation with a pelvic belt. The anesthetist has to take account of the position-induced pressure rise in the thorax when planning his anesthetic regimen.

---

*Patient Preparation for Laparoscopy*

---

Information
Evaluation of ability to undergo anesthesia
Cleaning and disinfection of umbilical fossa
(povidone-iodine swab)
Nasogastric tube
One-time catheterization

# Indications

## Diagnostic Laparoscopy

The increased use of laparoscopic techniques and growing expertise in their application justify the more liberal employment of diagnostic laparoscopy in abdominal surgery.

## Oncological Problems

Exploratory laparoscopy yields information on the extent of organ involvement or distant metastases of gastrointestinal tumors. Tissue samples for histological study can be collected by laparoscopy from tumors of the abdominal organs, suspect portions of the liver, and the peritoneum. Diagnostic laparoscopy can supply important criteria for decision-making on the local and general operability of intra-abdominal neoplasms. It also permits verification of the results of previous surgical, radiological, or cytostatic therapy. In individual cases, laparoscopy can obviate the need for exploratory laparotomy (Cuschieri 1980; Shandall and Johnson 1985).

## Evaluation of Atypical Abdominal Symptoms

Advances in diagnostic techniques such as imaging procedures and the sophistication of clinical chemistry tests have markedly reduced the incidence of unexplained abdominal symptoms. There remains a group of patients who defy definitive diagnosis in spite of all the imaging tests or endoluminal endoscopic investigations. Laparoscopy can be helpful in such cases. In the assessment of late local sequelae after abdominal operations, laparoscopy makes it possible to verify or rule out the presence of adhesions. The rate of success of laparoscopy in diagnosing unexplained abdominal complaints is generally reported to be 87.0−93.7% (Saleh 1978; Barry et al. 1978).

## Laparoscopic Appendectomy

The diagnosis of acute appendicitis remains one of the most difficult tasks in surgery. According to the literature, the rate of erroneous diagnoses varies between 10% and 20% (deDombal 1979). The hope that nonindicated appendectomies may be prevented or at least reduced in number by laparoscopy, that is, by a goal-oriented search and direct visual examination of a potentially pathological appendix, has not so far been realized to the desired extent. This is partly due to the fact that appendicitis begins in the mucosa and can cause clinical symptoms at a time when direct inspection of the serosa is not certain to uncover macroscopic alterations.

This puts the diagnostic value of laparoscopy in perspective in cases of suspected acute appendicitis. Laparoscopy nevertheless seems justified to us when it is performed for the purpose of evaluating clinically suspect findings. A strong argument in its favor is the opportunity it provides to perform laparoscopic appendectomy. If the clinical diagnosis is confirmed, the transition from diagnosis to treatment can be made immediately.

In the presence of a grossly unremarkable or only slightly altered appendix, the peritoneal cavity can be explored to look for other causes of the clinical picture and possibly identify their location (e.g., endometriosis, Meckel's diverticulum) without significant trauma to the abdominal organs. If no other pathological changes are detectable, the appendix should be laparoscopically removed, even in the absence of significant macroscopic findings.

Whether chronic or recurrent appendicitis is a valid indication for appendectomy remains questionable at this time. The extent to which this poorly understood disease can be clarified by systematic laparoscopy in suspected cases remains to be determined. There is no doubt that rare diseases, such as carcinoid and mucocele of the appendix can be discovered only by appendectomy early on. On the other hand, the sound and cosmetically attractive approach via laparoscopy does not excuse the removal of a healthy appendix.

If a perforated appendix or a perityphlitic abscess is found intraoperatively, it is up to the experienced surgeon to decide whether to proceed with the operation laparoscopically. As a rule, the conventional procedure is preferable. How to use the laparoscopic technique if there is good visualization and appropriate experience will be shown in the following chapters.

## Laparoscopic Cholecystectomy

The indication for cholecystectomy is not changed by the laparoscopic technique. The aim of this procedure is the same as that of the conventional operation, that is, removal of the diseased gallbladder. The ease of the technique and the cosmetically attractive, minimally involved procedure of laparoscopic cholecystectomy ought not to be an inducement for an untenable extension of the indication. As with the conventional procedure, the operation is indicated if the following criteria are satisfied:

– Symptomatic cholecystolithiasis
– Acute cholecystitis with cholelithiasis within the 72-h limit (at present advisable only for experienced surgeons)
– Asymptomatic cholelithiasis with threatened complication, e.g. due to multiple small calculi (danger of calculus migration), a large solitary stone (danger of mural necrosis), and sharp-edged chalk stones (chronic cholecystitis)
– Asymptomatic cholelithiasis in postendoscopic papillotomy (EPT) state
– The operation is also indicated in the presence of a non-visualizing cholecystogram (closure of cystic duct) and in diabetics tendency to inflammation!)

If the intraoperative cholangiogram should reveal an unsuspected common duct stone, laparoscopic choledochotomy with extraction of the stone and insertion of a T-drain is possible. However, this technique demands a high degree of expertise and experience on the part of the surgeon. It therefore cannot be generally recommended as yet and should at present be performed only by surgeons truly experienced, in the more intricate laparoscopic techniques. As an alternative approach in the treatment of common duct stones, postoperative endoscopic retrograde cholangiopancreatography (ERCP) with stone extraction is perfectly acceptable.

---

*Indications for Laparoscopy*

---

*Diagnostic:*

    Oncology:
        tumor staging
        collection of tissue samples
        monitoring of therapy

    Differential diagnosis:
        atypical abdominal symptoms
        pain in the right lower abdomen
        "adhesion complaints"

*Therapeutic:*

    Acute appendicitis
    Acute cholecystitis
    Symptomatic cholelithiasis,
    Asymptomatic cholelithiasis with
        threatened complications
    Asymptomatic cholelithiasis in post-EPT
        state
    Adhesions

# Contraindications

## General Contraindications to Laparoscopy

Since laparoscopy causes the patient little discomfort and is associated with a low rate of complications, the indications for it can be defined broadly. Still, general contraindications specific for the method need to be taken into consideration.

## Cardiorespiratory Disorders

Preoperatively extant all are cardiac and pulmonary conditions which may lead to restricted respiratory function and/or possible cardiac function disorders in the presence of a pneumoperitoneum. These are: decompensated heart failure, cardiac conduction defects, recent myocardial infarction, and severe obstructive pulmonary disease. Compensated cardiac failure as well as stable angina pectoris are not absolute contraindications.

## Blood Coagulation Disorders

Inasmuch as laparoscopy is most often an elective procedure, the presence of a coagulation disorder requires the institution of appropriate treatment or replacement therapy and postponement of the operation until correction of the defective coagulation factors has been achieved. Refractory coagulation disorders, however, should be regarded as absolute contraindications to laparoscopic surgery.

## Ileus

Air- and fluid-filled intestinal loops in patients with mechanical or paralytic ileus pose the risk of an accidental injury to a hollow and thin-walled viscus during induction of the pneumoperitoneum. From an absolute contraindication in the hands of the novice, they have become an experience-related contraindication in the hands of a seasoned laparoscopic surgeon.

## Infections

Abdominal wall infections are a contraindication because of the risk of intra-abdominal dissemination of pathogenic microorganisms and the creation of a generalized peritonitis.

## Obesity, Diaphragmatic Hernia

With the development of extra-long trocars and corresponding Verres needles, laparoscopy is no longer contraindicated in extremely obese patients. They do benefit from the minimal approach routes of the laparoscopic procedure. Nor is diaphragmatic hernia a contraindication anymore. The occurrence of a pneumomediastinum in patients with large diaphragmatic hernias can be prevented by Trendelenburg positioning (15°), limitation of the intra-abdominal pressure to 10 mmHg, and endotracheal anesthesia.

## Contraindications to Laparoscopic Appendectomy

The choice of the laparoscopic procedure is only made intraoperatively, depending on the local findings. Phlegmons of the cecal wall in the area of the base of the appendix are a contraindication to the laparoscopic procedure, as is perforation of the appendix near the base, unless instruments are available to include safely and aseptically the involved walls of the cecal cul-de-sac with the appendiceal specimen, e.g., the linear closing and cutting stapler.

If the base of the appendix cannot be clearly exposed, exploration by open laparotomy is preferable to laparoscopic removal.

A carcinoid near the base of the appendix, like an appendiceal carcinoma, usually cannot be radically removed by laparoscopic appendectomy alone.

## Contraindications to Laparoscopic Cholecystectomy

As in appendectomy, the decision in favor of laparoscopic removal of the gallbladder is generally made intraoperatively. The following are preoperative contraindications: acute pancreatitis, confirmed choledocholithiasis with obstructive jaundice, and suspected gallbladder or bile ducts carcinoma. Acute cholecystitis as well as a previous upper abdominal operation are no longer contraindications for those experienced in laparoscopy. The intraoperative findings will be the determining factor.

The following are the principal intraoperative contraindications: perforation of the gallbladder with biliary peritonitis, inflammation of the hepatoduodenal ligament, and a gallbladder that is directly attached to the common bile duct. If the intraoperative cholangiography should unexpectedly disclose a choledochal calculus, cholecystectomy alone should be performed, particularly in elderly patients. The stone extraction is carried out later by ERCP. In young patients, choledochotomy and stone extraction are performed in the same session, either via laparoscopy or via laparotomy, depending on the surgeon's experience.

All in all, results obtained with laparoscopic operative techniques to date warrant caution in the interpretation of indications and contraindications. It may be taken as a general rule that the decision must depend on the laparoscopist's experience and his or her overall surgical expertise. Rigid guidelines would be neither helpful nor realistic at the present time since everything is in flux in this field of active methodological development. A good rule to observe is that circumspection and recourse to established procedures are a safe high ground on which to stand rather than to be motivated by an over-enthusiastic pioneering spirit and lack of a critical perspective.

---

*Contraindications to Laparoscopy*

---

*General:*

    Cardiorespiratory disorders
    Refractory coagulation disorders
    Ileus
    Abdominal wall infections
    Generalized peritonitis

*Specific:*
For appendectomy

    Phlegmons of the cecal wall and
        perforation near the base
        (depending on experience and
        availability of specialized instruments)
    Carcinoid near base of appendix
    Carcinoma of appendix

For cholecystectomy:

    Perforation of the gallbladder
    Acute pancreatitis
    Obstructive jaundice due to
        choledocholithiasis,
    Mirizzi's syndrome

---

# Anesthesia

For diagnostic and operative laparoscopy, anesthesia may be local, regional, by face-mask, and through an endotracheal tube. The choice of the method of anesthesia for diagnostic laparoscopy has been influenced largely by the available facilities. However, in operative laparoscopic surgery, general anesthesia with endotracheal intubation, muscle relaxation, and controlled ventilation is preferred. This is due to the involvement of the pain-sensitive peritoneum and the need for a lasting pneumoperitoneum. The advantages are deeper sedation and relaxation, which help in the performance of protracted, delicate manipulations. There also is the opportunity of changing over to laparotomy at any time.

The cardiorespiratory monitoring customarily practiced during general anesthesia permits the early detection and control of incipient complications. This applies especially to the reported decrease of cardiac output (Brantley and Riley 1988; Lee 1975; Motew et al. 1973) and the onset of bradycardic arrhythmias in 5–10% of cases (Wurst and Finsterer 1990). Typical side effects of laparoscopy, such as a reduction of compliance of the chest wall and elevation of the diaphragm upon a rise in intra-abdominal pressure above 12 mmHg, are associated with an ensuing decrease of respiratory volume, acidosis, and tachycardia. These should be as familiar to the anesthetist as the measures necessary fot their treatment.

With a prolonged $CO_2$ pneumoperitoneum in particular, adjustment of the respiratory volume is needed in the exchange of the individually varying amounts of $CO_2$ gas via the pulmonary alveoli. Induction of the pneumoperitoneum with $CO_2$ gas under general anesthesia and mechanical ventilation is associated with a rise of 10 mmHg in the arterial carbon dioxide pressure.

The reported high rate of postoperative nausea and vomiting, ranging up to 50% (Hovorka et al. 1989; Brown et al. 1984), following laparoscopy is probably attributable less to the selected anesthetic regimen than to other factors (Kurer and Welch 1984; Skacel et al. 1986; Kenefick et al. 1987).

# Technique of Laparoscopic Procedures

## Diagnostic Laparoscopy

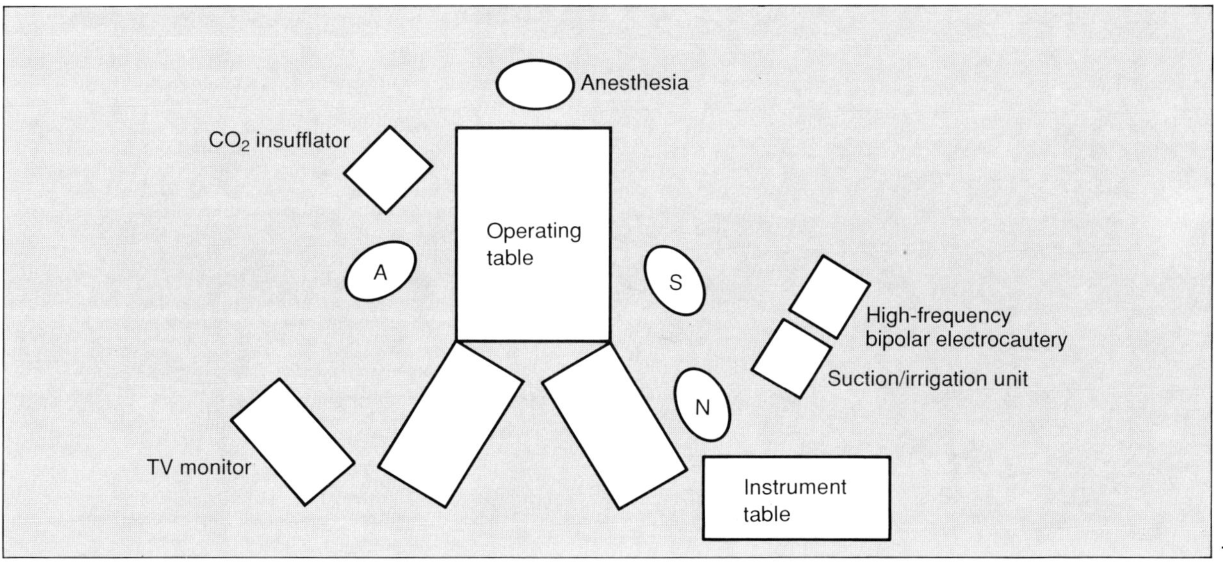


**13**

### Disposition of Equipment and Position of Surgical Team
(Fig. **13**)

- Surgeon (S), on the patient's left

- Assistant (A), on the patient's right

- Surgical nurse (N) and instrument table at the foot and left side of the patient

- TV monitor and $CO_2$ insufflator at patient's right side within the surgeon's angle of vision; these instruments may be separated, as shown here, or superimposed at the right leg of the patient, facilitating the surgeon's line of vision and work in the same direction

- Manipulation of camera by surgeon or by assistant

Optional: A second video monitor at the left shoulder of the patient will make the assistant's task much easier.

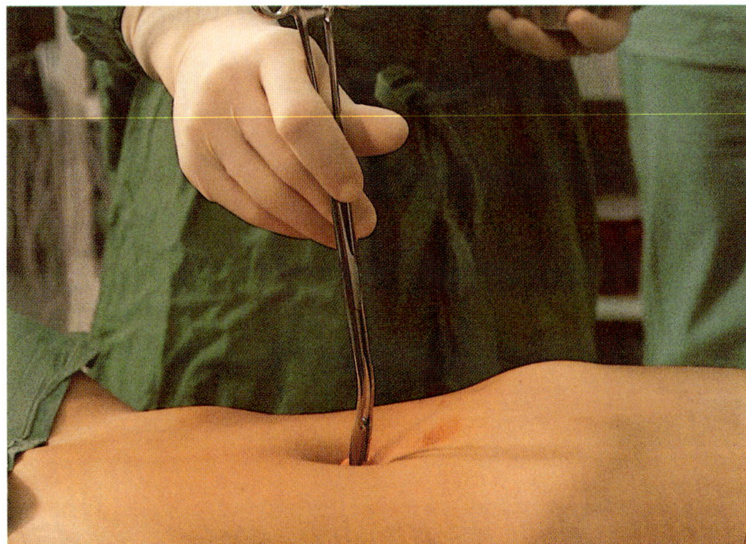

**Preparation and Insertion of Verres Needle**
(Figs. **14–16**)

– Sterile draping of operative field
– Disinfection of abdominal wall
– Cleansing of umbilical fossa with swab

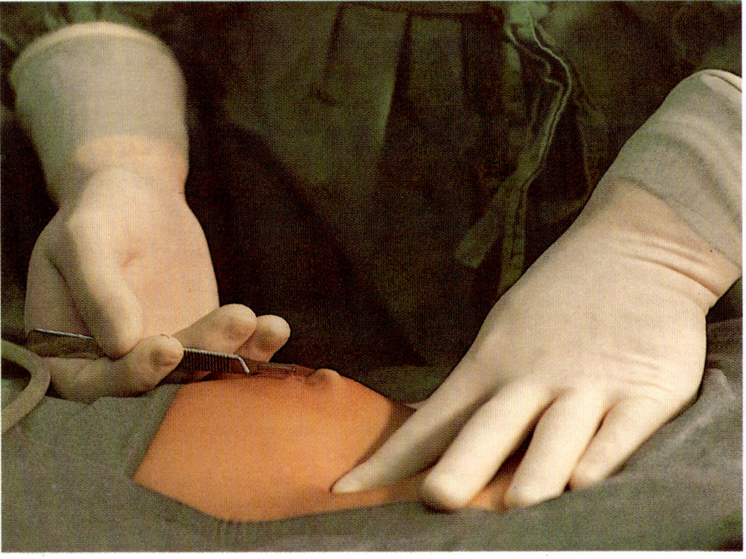

– Incision of skin at inferior border of umbilicus with pointed scalpel
– Check on function of Verres needle (snap mechanism, patency)

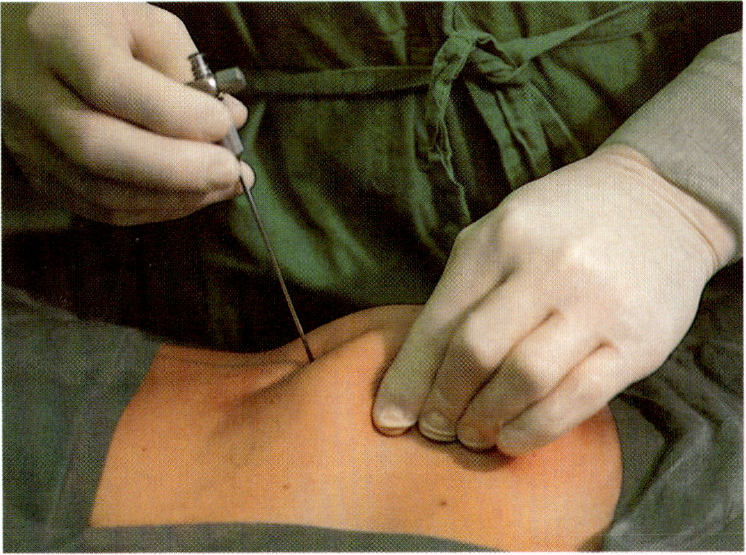

– Elevation of abdominal wall with the left hand
– Vertical insertion of the Verres needle through the abdominal wall layers. The needle is held steady with the propped-up little finger of the right hand. The entry into the free abdominal cavity is audible as the snap mechanism is activated

## Safety Test
(Figs. **17–19**)

- Application of a syringe containing 10 ml of saline solution; resistance-free injection of the liquid and attempt at aspiration

- Aspiration of blood or intestinal contents; retraction of needle and new attempt at puncture or, in the presence of adhesions (history!), possibly minilaparotomy

- Aspiration of air bubbles indicates a correct position of the needle

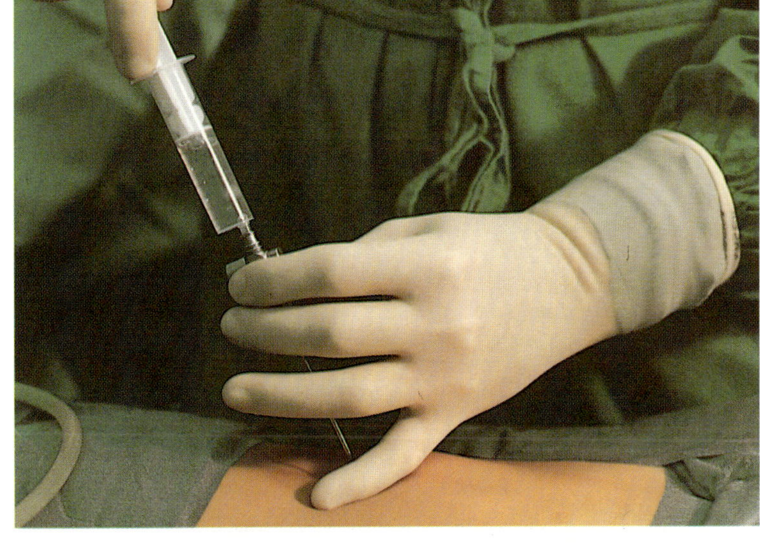

- Slurp test: Physiological saline solution is instilled into the needle and the abdominal wall is raised; if the solution runs freely into the peritoneum, the needle is in the right position

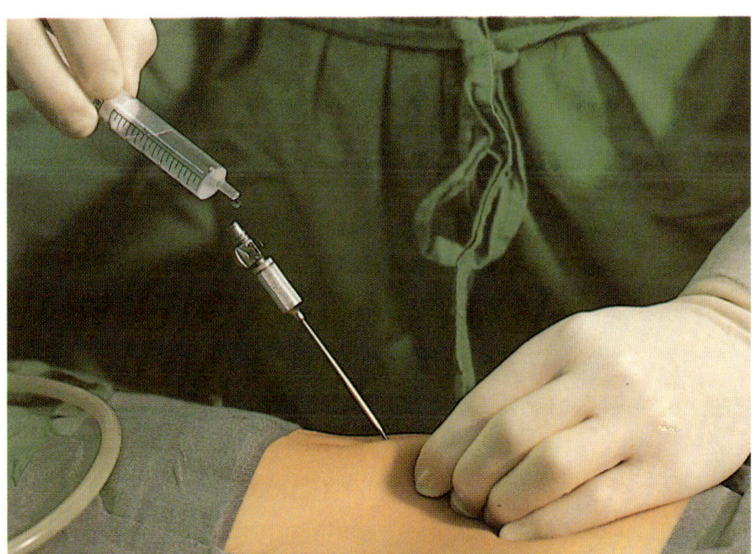

- Start of gas insufflation, initially at a low flow rate (1 l/min)

- Constant flow and intra-abdominal pressures up to a maximum of 10 mmHg are also indicative of correct placement of the needle in the abdominal cavity

- The abdominal cavity is filled up at the maximal flow rate (6 l/min) under electronic control. *Beware of asymmetrical elevation of the abdominal wall = insufflation of hollow organs!*

- Meanwhile, pending production of the desired intra-abdominal pressure (10–12 mmHg in children and 12–14 mmHg in adults), the video camera, the light cable, the scope, etc. are installed

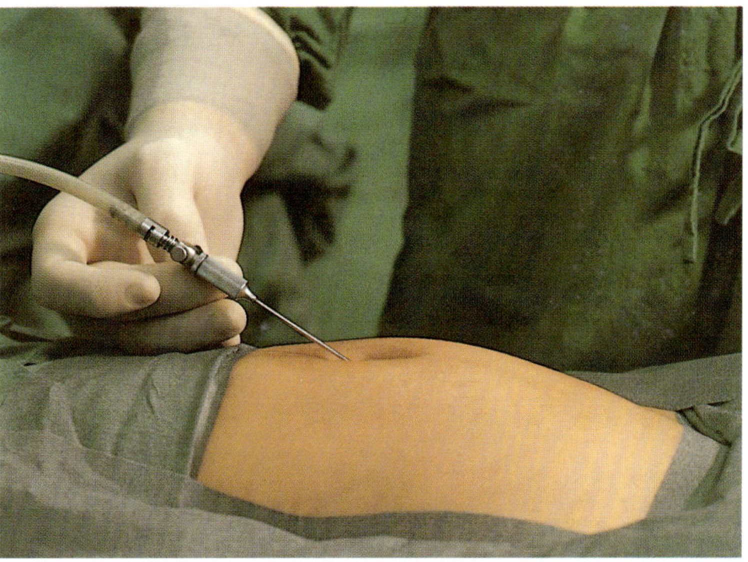

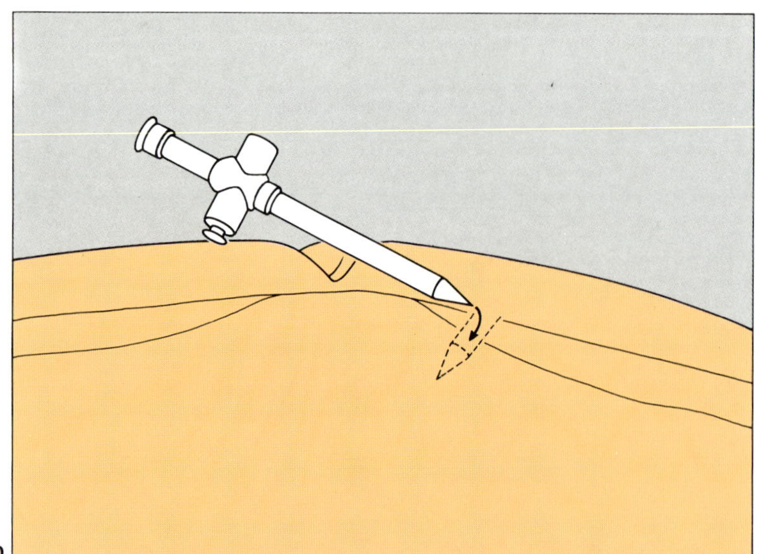

## Placement of Laparoscopic Trocar (LT)
(Figs. **20—24**)

– Insertion of the conically shaped trocar by the Semm Z-puncture technique *(watch for epigastric vessels!)*

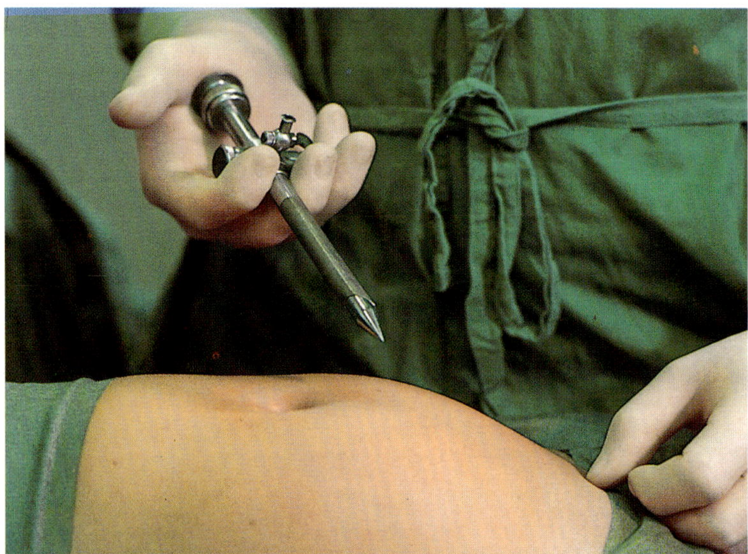

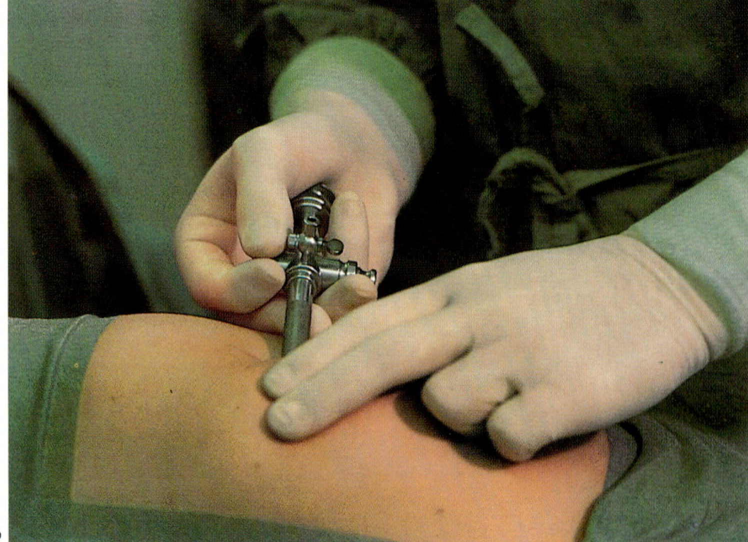

– First, the trocar is passed about 2—4 cm subcutaneously in the horizontal plane in a lateral direction

– For deeper penetrations, the abdominal wall is slightly raised and the right hand is steadied against the trocar by the little finger. The movement is from the wrist in the direction of the pelvis

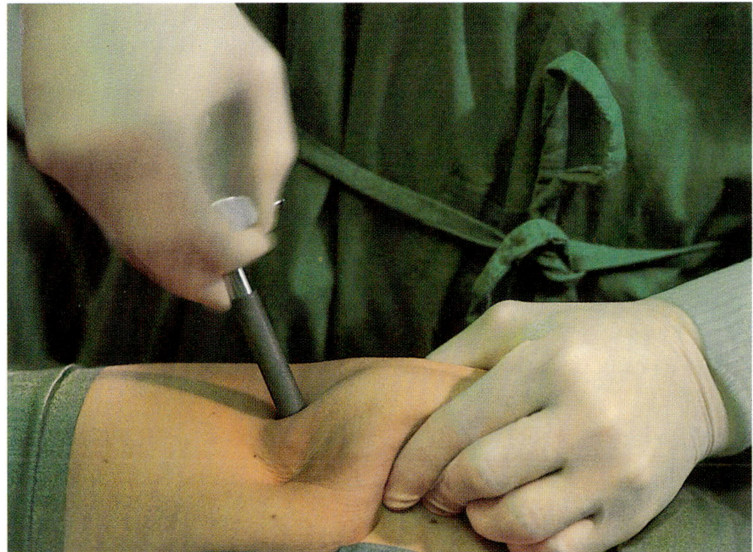

23

– After penetration of the abdominal wall, the trocar is pulled out, and the laparoscope is advanced into the sheath, and the gas tube is attached

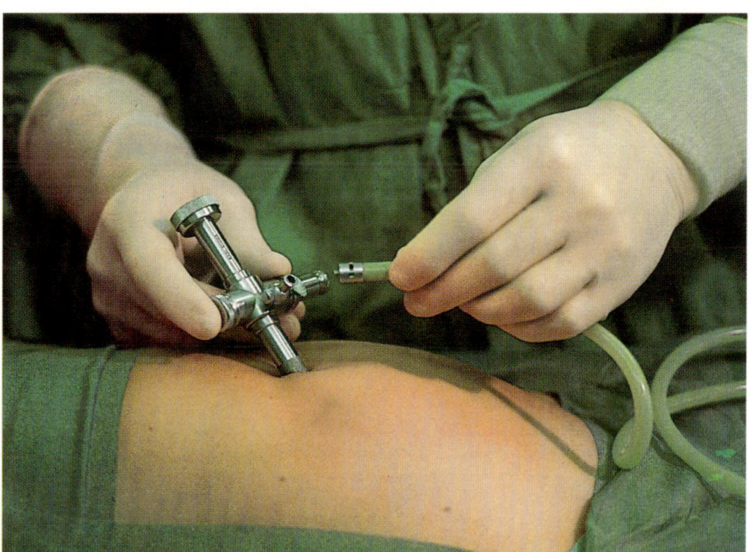

24

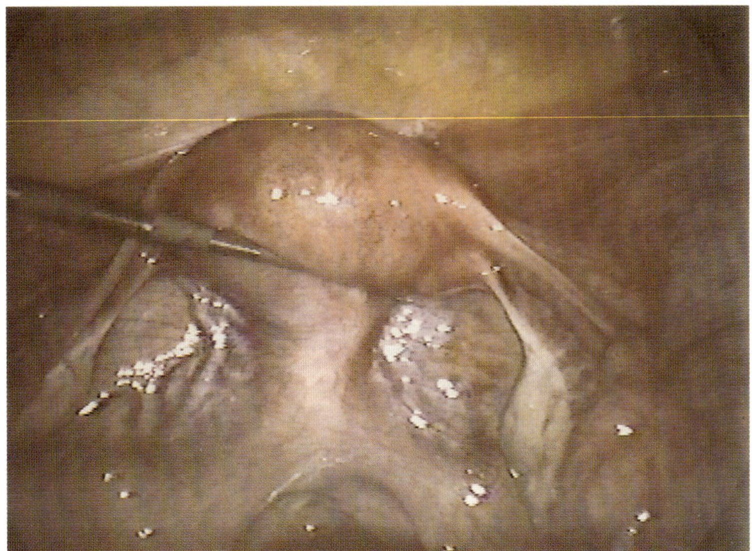

25

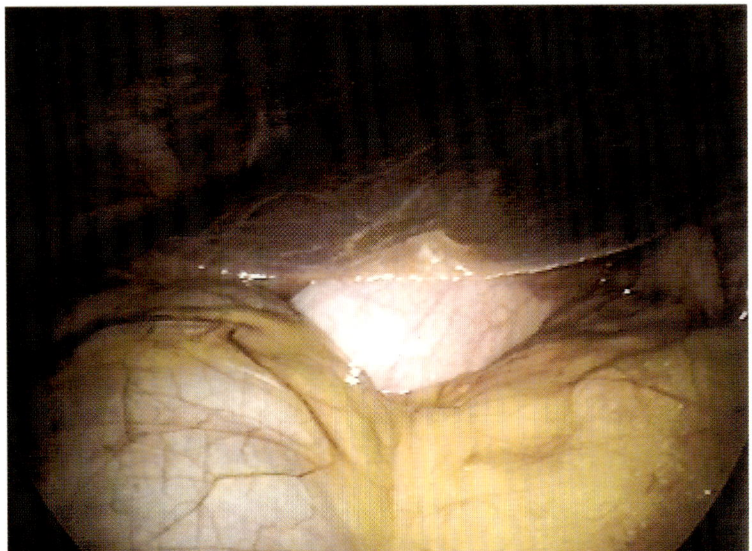

26

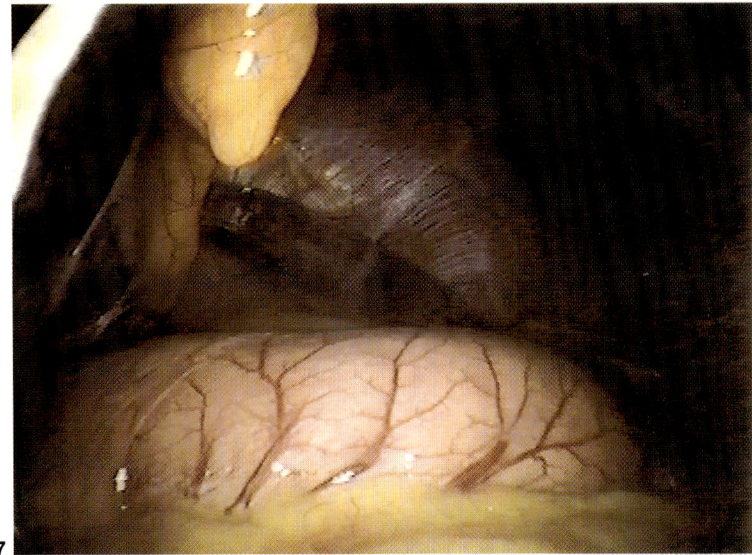

27

## Visual Diagnostic Exploration
(Figs. **25–27**)

- Orientational 360° examination
- Injuries due to the Verres needle or the trocar are ruled out (free blood? intestinal secretions? retroperitoneal hematoma?)
- Evaluation of visible organs
- Evaluation of operability

## Placement of Operating Trocars (OT)
(Figs. **28−30**)

– Localization according to proposed operation

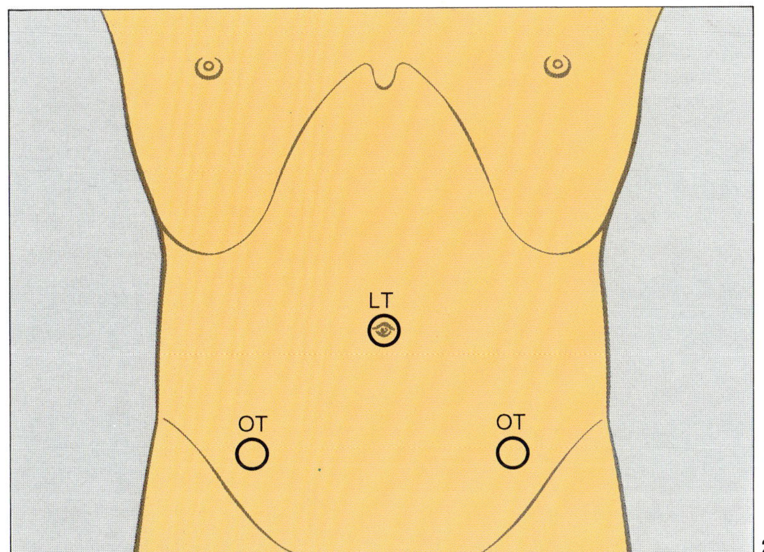


– Selection of an avascular site by transillumination

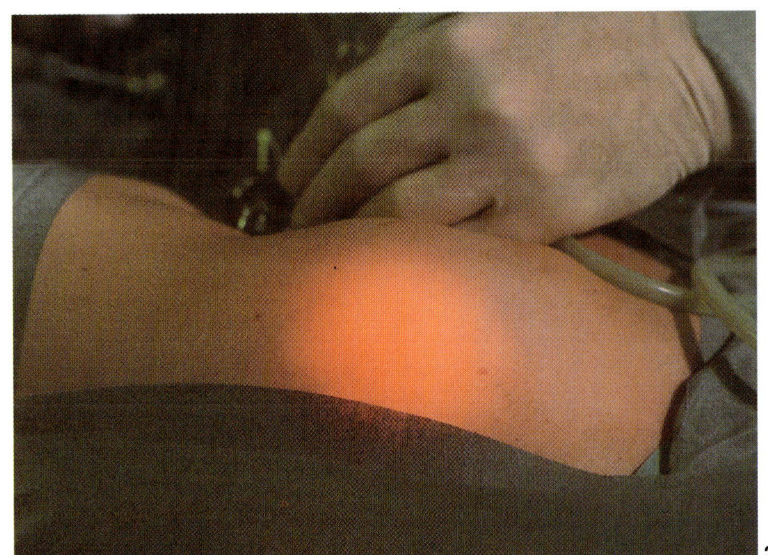

– Penetration into the peritoneum under endoscopic vision
– Performance of the planned operation

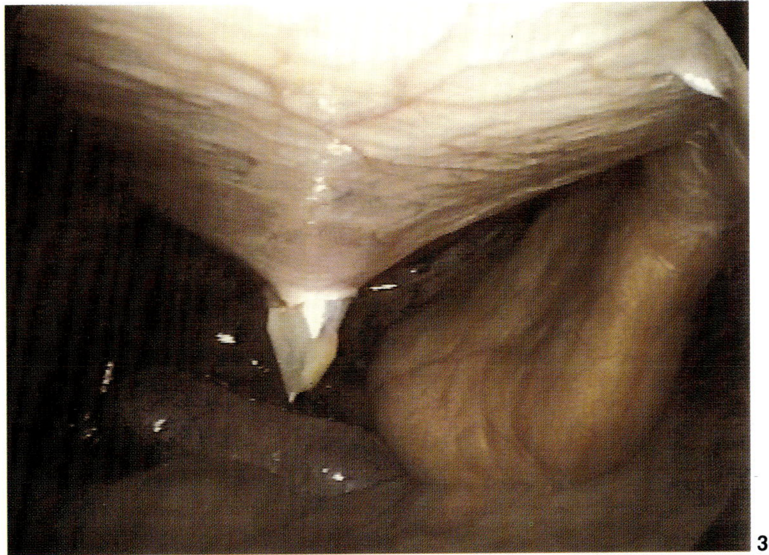

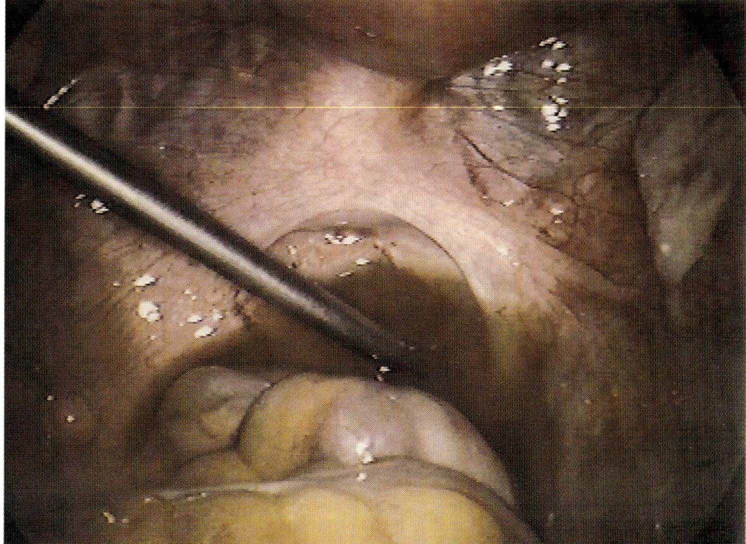

**31**

## Conclusion of Laparoscopy
(Figs. **31—33**)

- Inspection of operative site
- Inspection of the lowest point (e.g., cul-de-sac of Douglas, subphrenic space); possibly, aspiration of secretions; verification of correct position of drain if one was placed

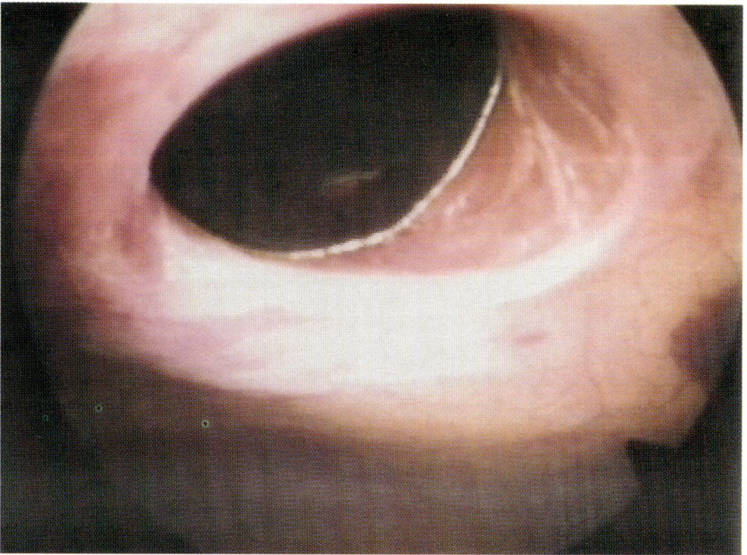

**32**

- Withdrawal of trocar sheaths under visual control
- *Beware of retraction of omentum and intestine into the incision site!*
- *Watch for bleeding from the puncture channel!*

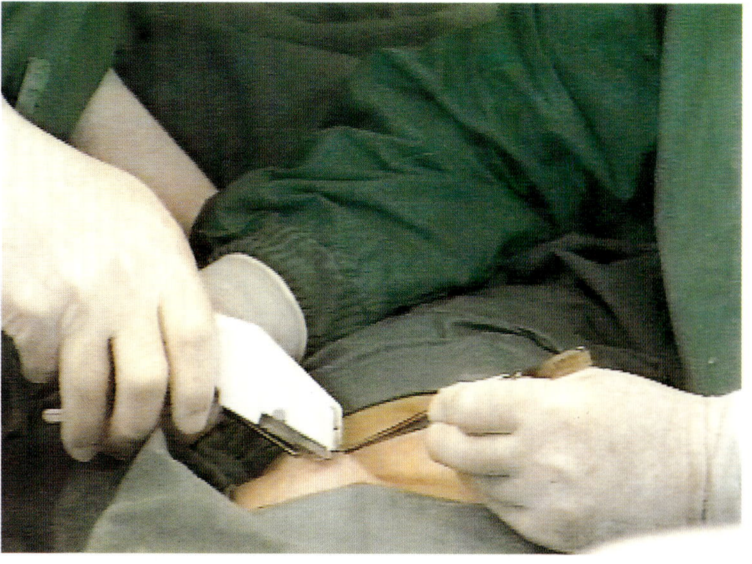

**33**

- After withdrawal of the laparoscope, the pneumoperitoneum is completely released through the open trocar sheath
- Suture of fascia for incisions $> 1$ cm
- Skin suture, sterile dressing

## Peritoneal Adhesions—Entry under Endoscopic Vision According to Semm
(Fig. **34 a–c**)

- Introduction of the laparoscopic trocar to the level of the musculature using the Z-puncture technique

- Exchange of trocar for laparoscope

- Penetration of the musculature by the laparoscope, under endoscopic visions, to the level of the peritoneum

- A white opaque surface indicates underlying adhesions

- Search for a free site in the peritoneum indicated by a dark, avascular surface using a rotating movement of the laparoscope over the deep fascia

- Following identification of a free area, the perforation is bluntly made with the elliptically shaped trocar sheath or after replacement of the laparoscope by the trocar

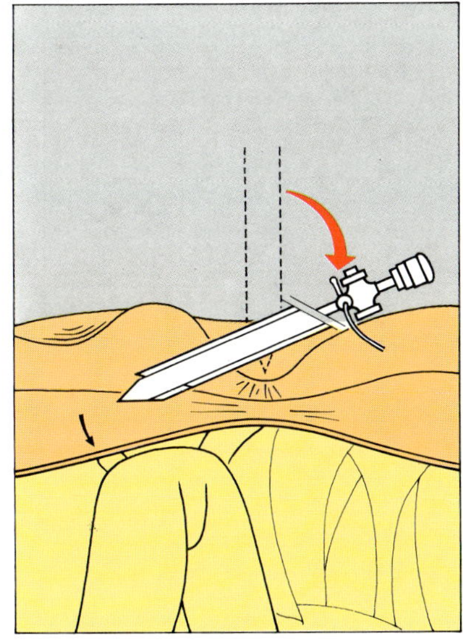
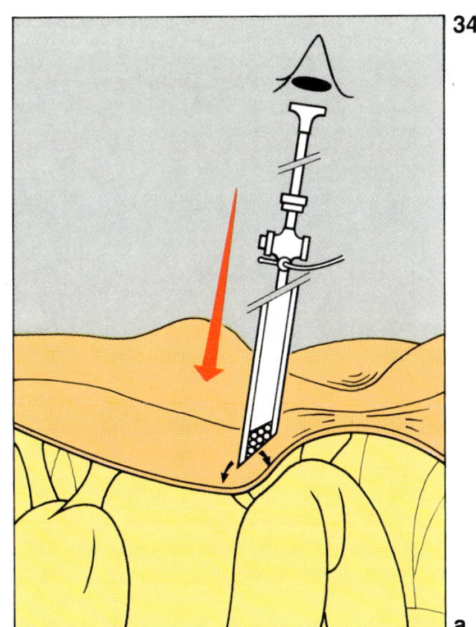

a

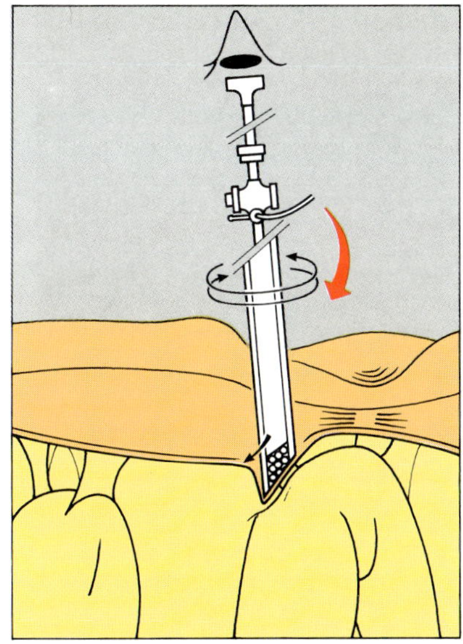
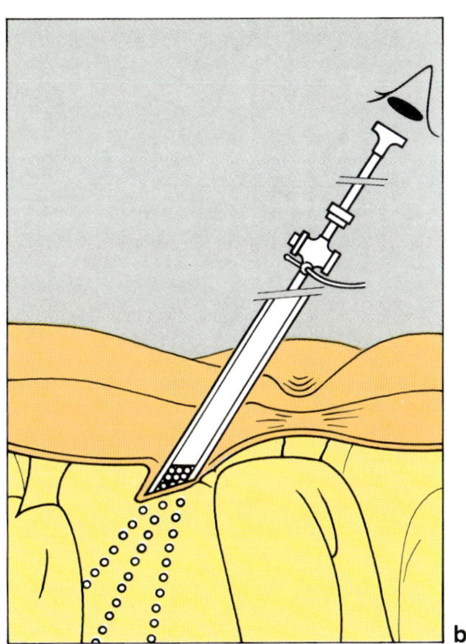

b

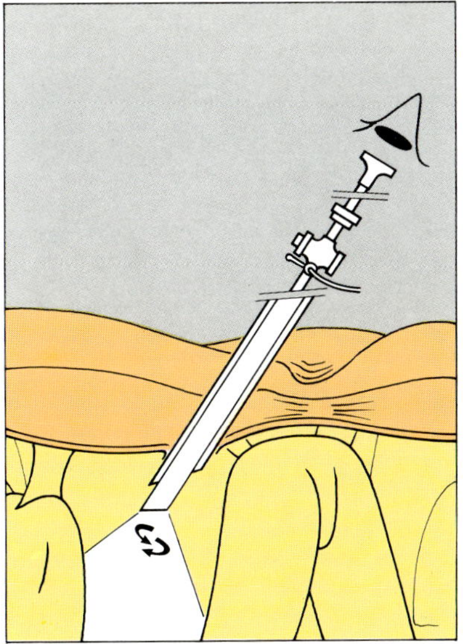
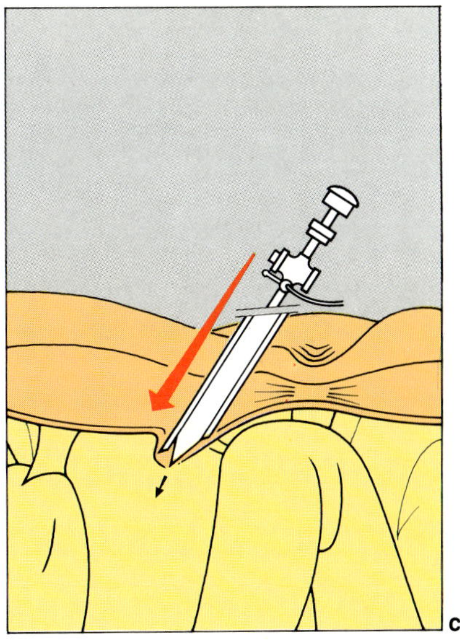

c

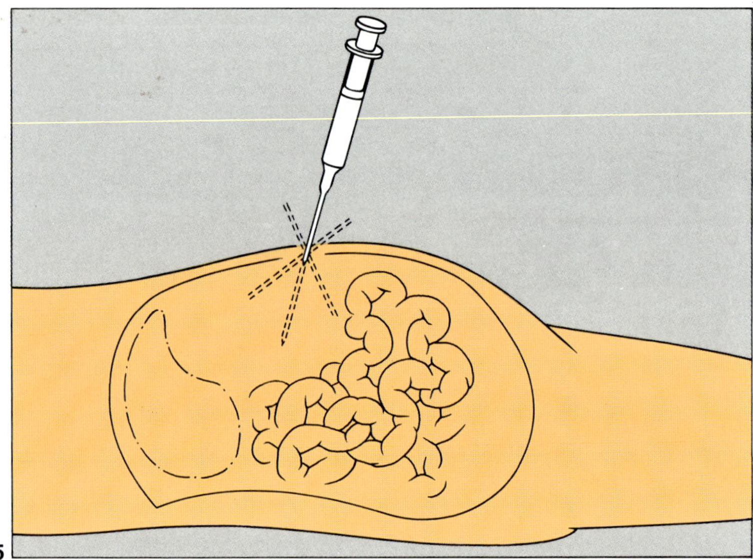

## Alternative Technique in Case of Peritoneal Adhesions
(Fig. **35**)

- The abdominal cavity is entered with the Verres needle in an area presumably free of adhesions (opposite the site of the previous operation)
- Aspiration test and 360° rotation of the needle in the abdomen to rule out adhesions in this area
- Induction of pneumoperitoneum
- Blind puncture with the laparoscopic trocar in the area of the puncture site

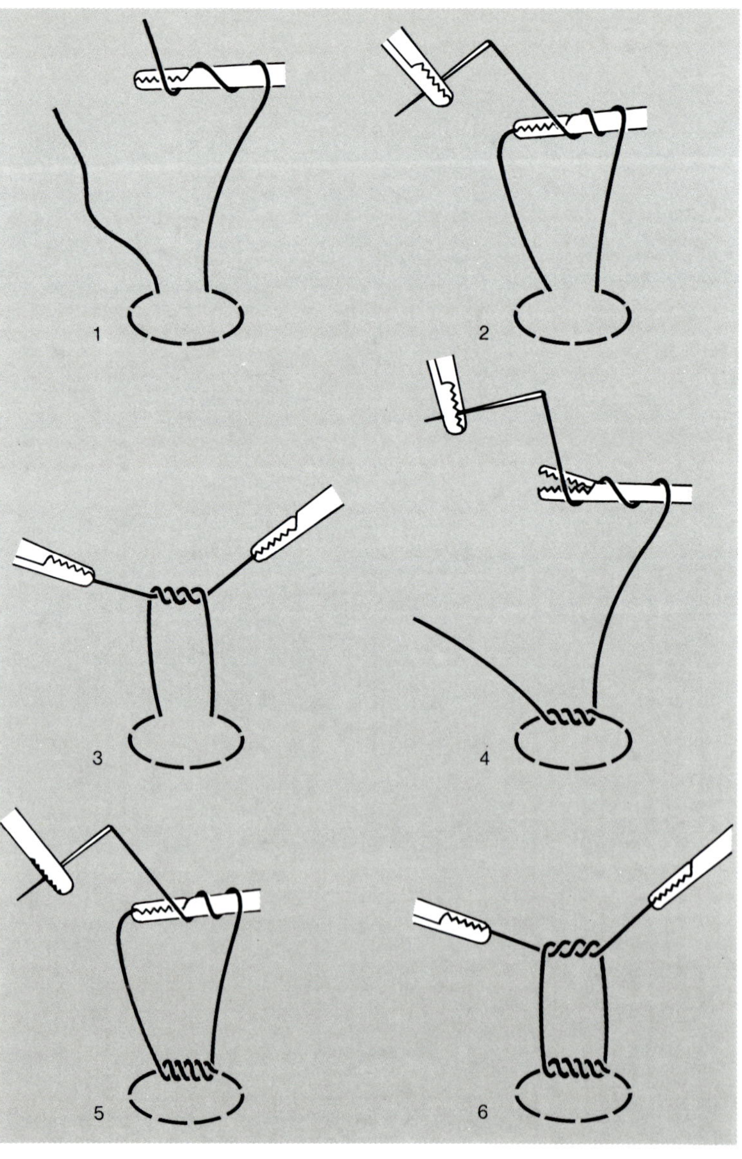

## Intra-abdominal Knot Tying
(Fig. **36**)

- Placement of needle and thread through a size reducer attached to the 11-mm operating trocar
- Inside the abdomen the needle is grasped with the needle holder, which has been introduced via a second, 5.5-mm operating trocar
- The free suture end is seized with a second needle holder placed through the first trocar, and a square surgical instrument knot is tied just as in open abdominal operations
- The knot is tightened by traction at both ends with the needle holders, and a second, reinforcing knot is tied
- The suture ends are cut with scissors
- The suture ends are extracted

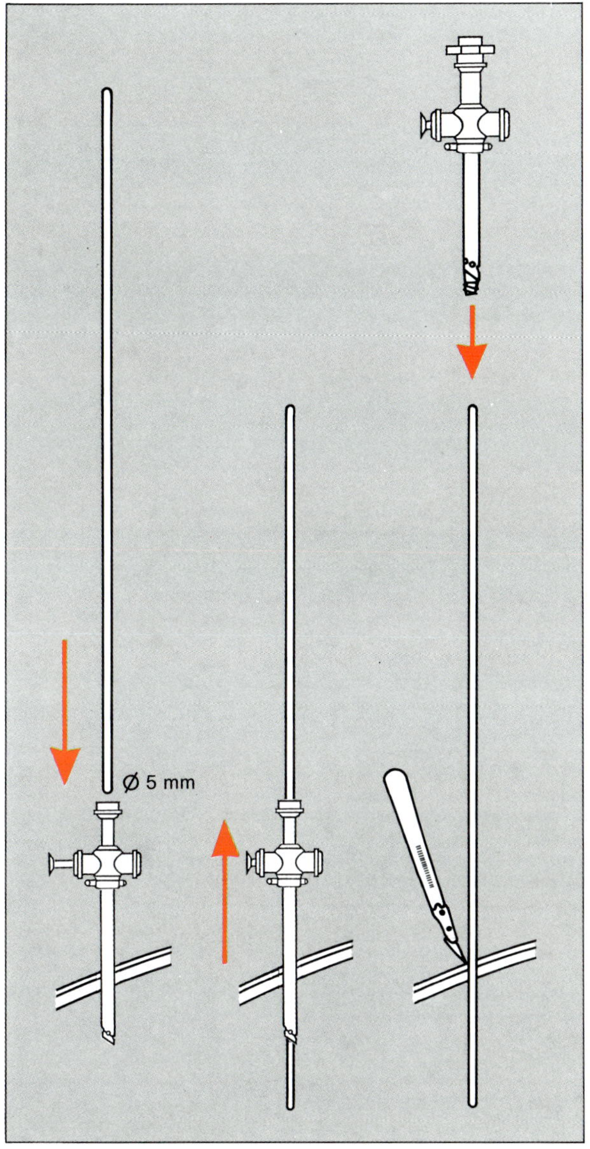

37a

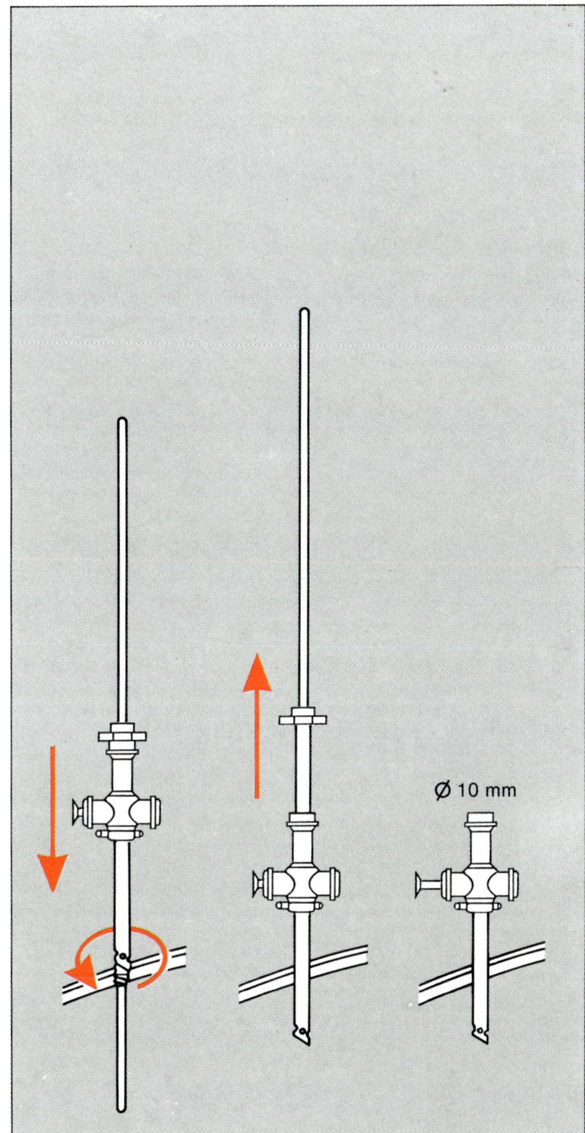

37b

## Exchange of Operating Trocar
(Fig. **37 a, b**)

- To hold the position, a guide rod is inserted through the trocar sheath
- The trocar sheath is withdrawn, and the skin incision is enlarged around the rod with a scalpel

- Insertion of threaded dilator with attached trocar sheath over the guide rod, using light pressure and rotary movements
- Withdrawal of guide rod and threaded dilator

# Appendectomy

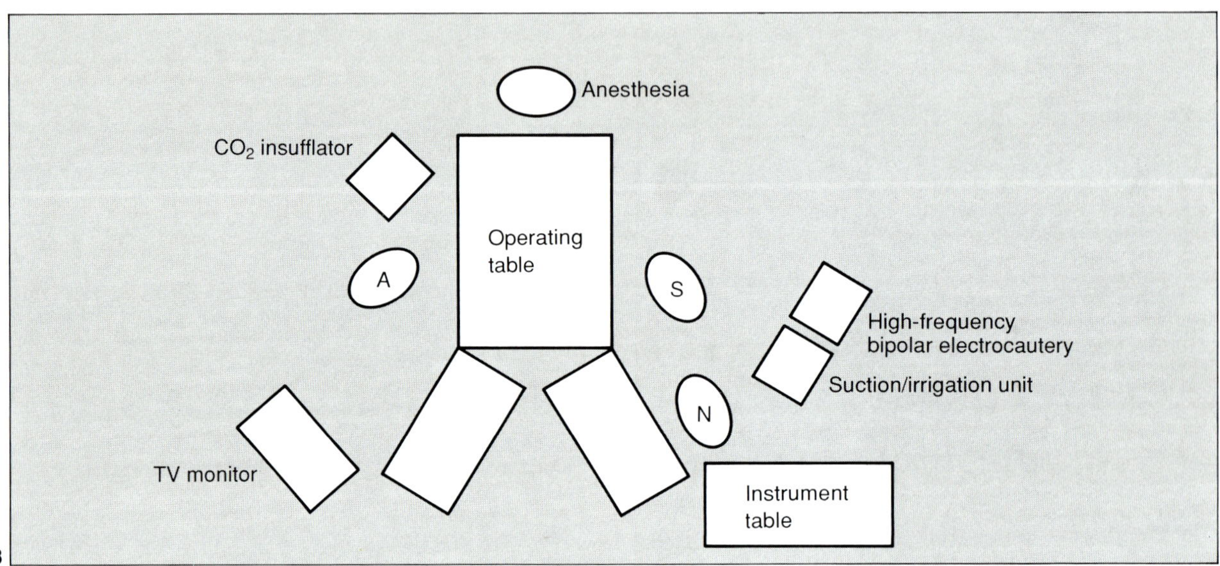


**38**

## Disposition of Equipment and Position of Surgical Team
(Fig. **38**)

- Surgeon (S) on the patient's left side
- Assistant (A) on the patient's right side
- Surgical nurse (N) and instrument table at the left foot end
- Monitor and $CO_2$ insufflator at the patient's right side in the surgeon's line of vision
- Manipulation of camera by surgeon

  Optional: A second video monitor at the left shoulder of the patient will make the assistant's task much easier.

## Placement of Trocar and Diagnostic Exploration
(Figs. **39–41**)

- Incision at the caudal umbilical margin (10 mm)

- Induction of pneumoperitoneum

- Insertion of an 11-mm trocar (7 mm in children) by the paramedian technique *(watch for epigastric vessels!)*

- Insertion of end-viewing laparoscope; diagnostic panoramic inspection

- Evaluation of operability

- Placement of operating trocars under endoscopic vision in the left and right lower abdomen with the aid of transillumination *(watch for epigastric vessels!)*

- A 5.5-mm trocar is placed in the left lateral lower abdomen at the level of the pubic hairline for the palpation probe, coagulation forceps, Roeder endoloop, and scissors

- Exploration of the lower abdominal organs with the palpation rod (ovary, fallopian tube, etc.) and identification of the appendix

- Insertion of a second operating trocar, 11 mm, in the right lateral lower abdomen at the level of the pubic hairline for appendix extraction and grasping forceps

- The table is tilted to the left (10°–20°) and the patient placed in head-down position (10°–20°)

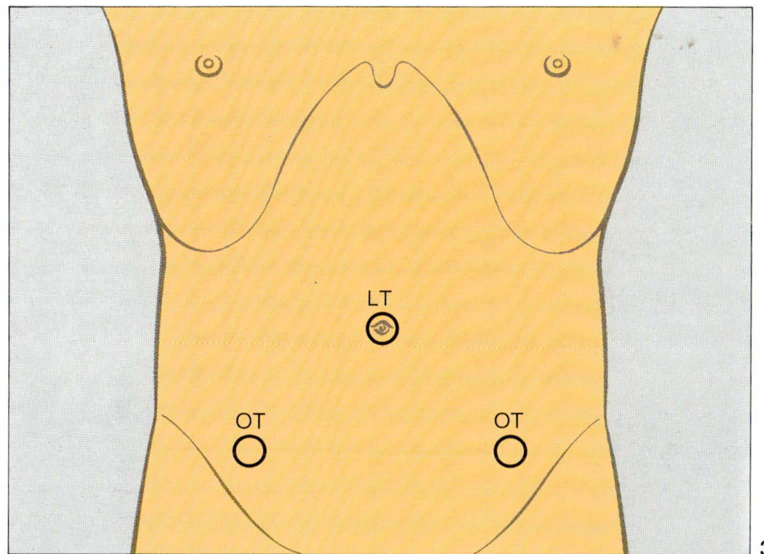


**39**

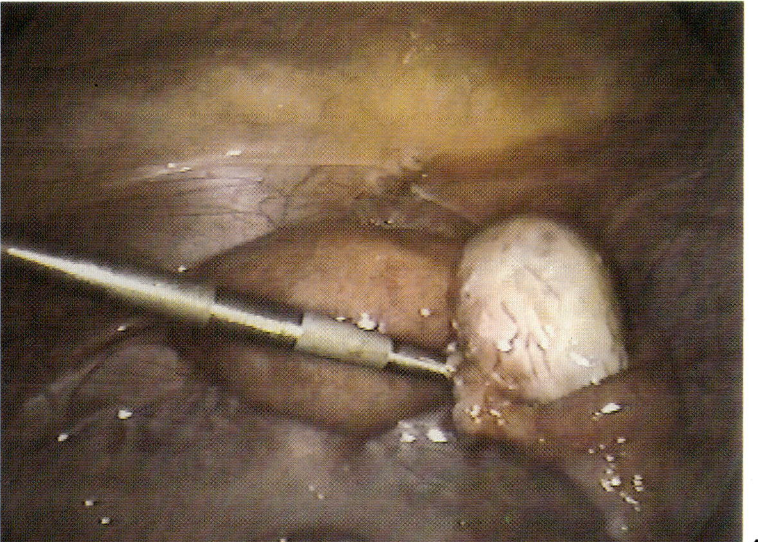

**40**

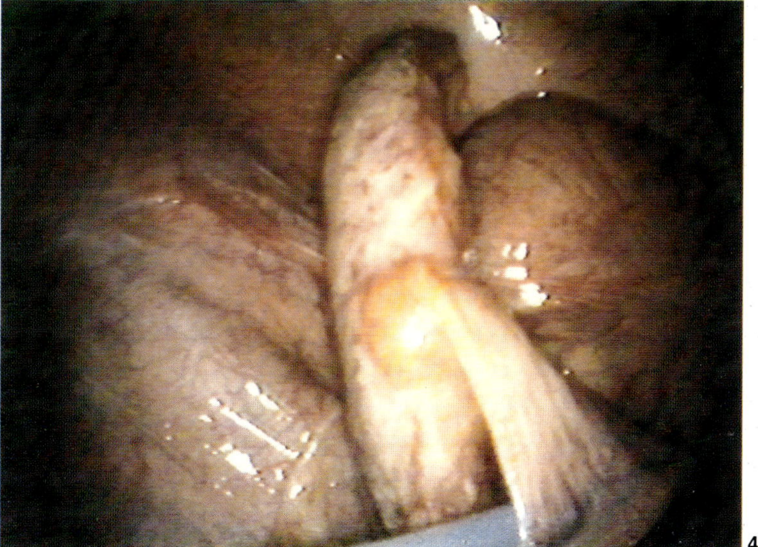

**41**

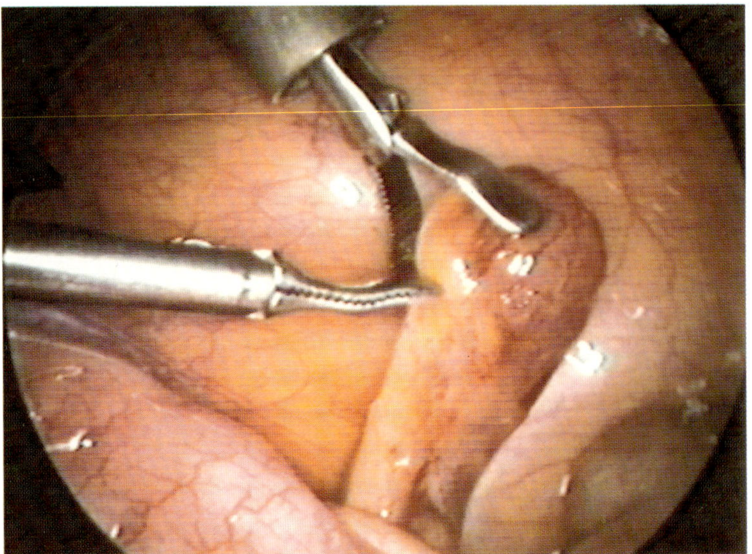

## Skeletization of Appendix
(Figs. **42—44**)

– Insertion of the atraumatic forceps, and grasping of appendiceal tip

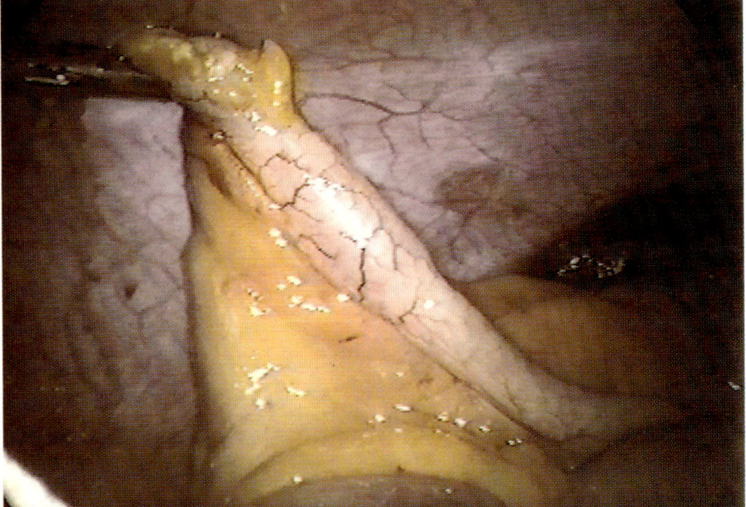

– The mesoappendix is stretched by raising the tip of the appendix toward the abdominal wall (assistant)

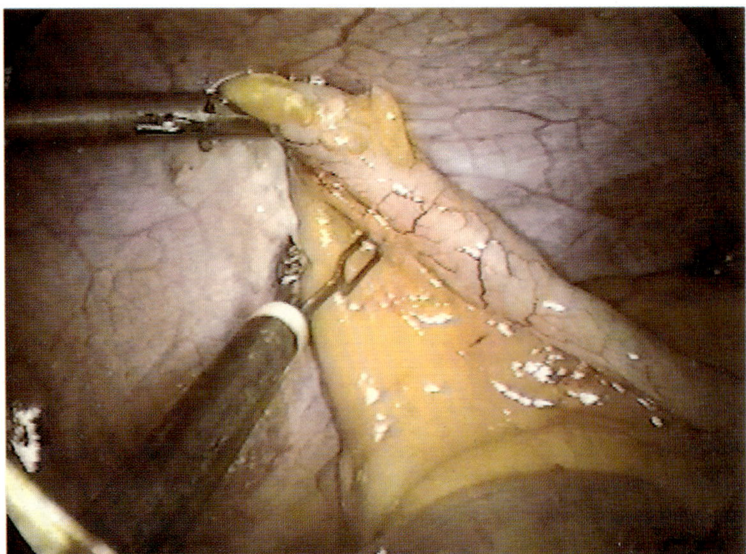

– Stepwise coagulation of the mesoappendix and the appendicular vessels with the bipolar forceps

(Figs. **45–47**)

– Stepwise division of coagulated
  areas with scissors

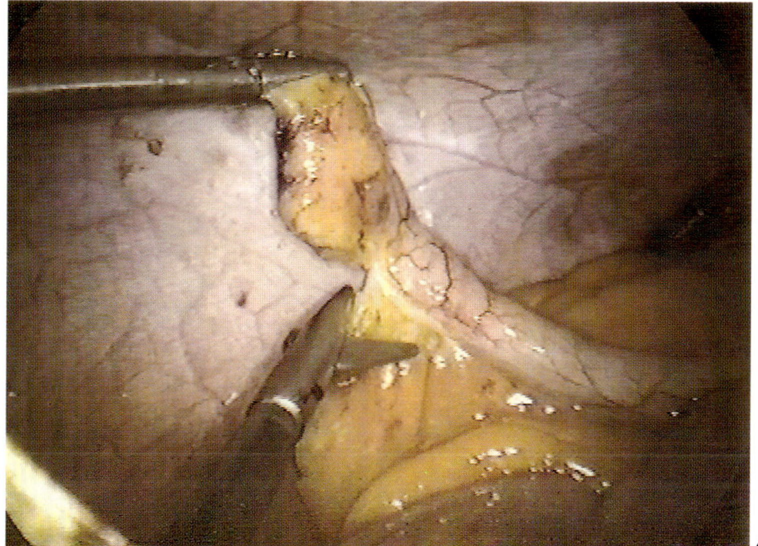

45

– Possible bleeding from the appendicular artery is controlled by coagulation with the bipolar forceps
– Fixation of the 5.5-mm trocar in
  place by the first assistant when re-
  placing instruments facilitates quick
  re-identification of the operative
  site

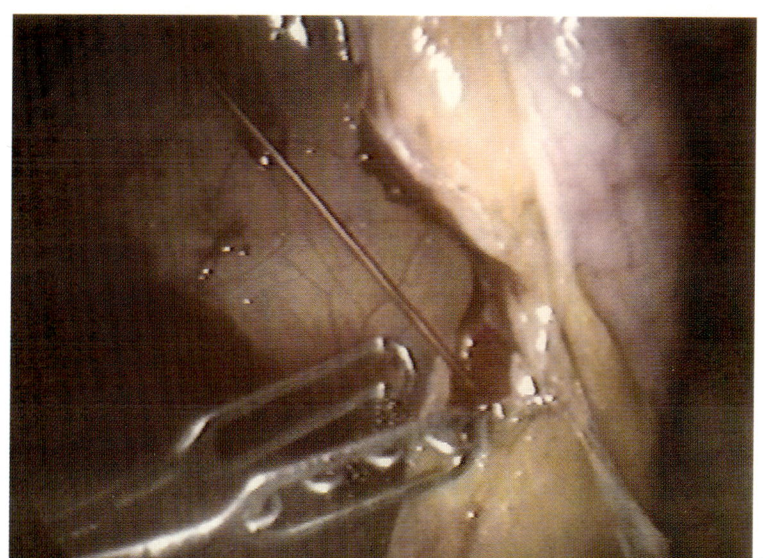

46

– The appendix is isolated to its base
  *(beware of coagulation of the cecal
  pole and terminal ileum!)*
– Stepwise withdrawal of the appendix
  into the extractor sheath
– Circular dissection of the base is required for ligation; additional adhesions are dissected free bluntly, or
  coagulated and sharply divided

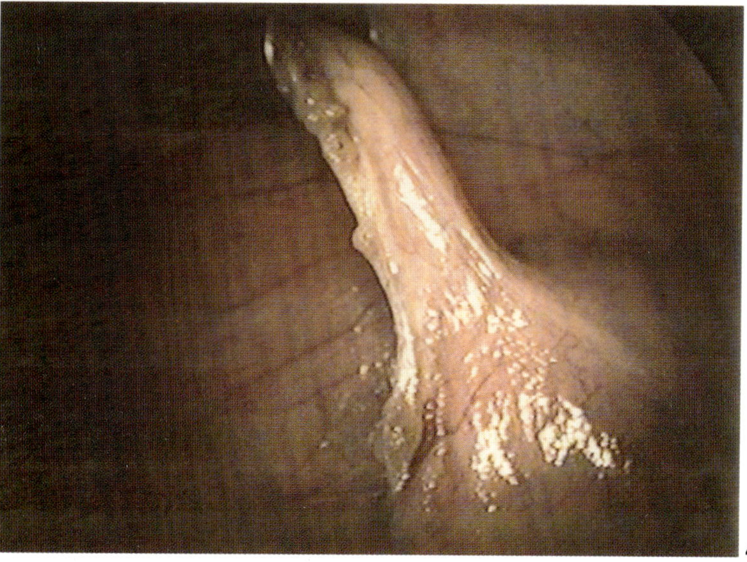

47

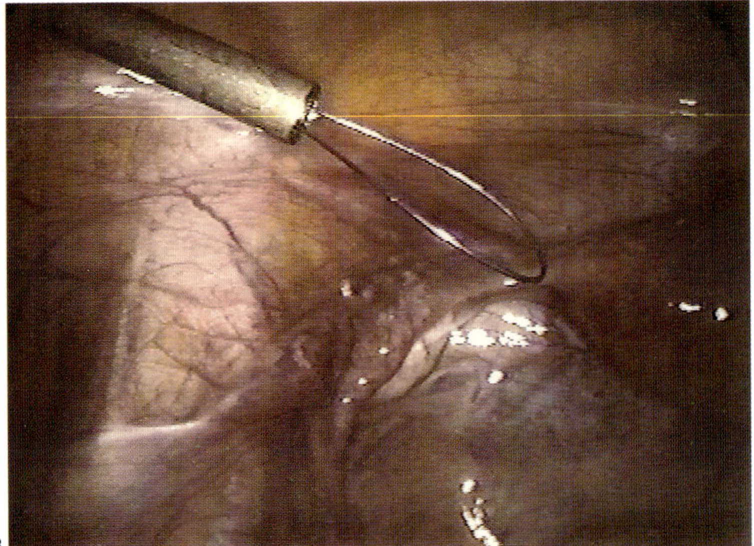

**48**

## Ablation of Appendix
(Figs. **48–56**)

- The isolated appendix is placed in the field of vision
- The loop applicator with the prepared Roeder endoloop is inserted through the 5.5-mm operating trocar

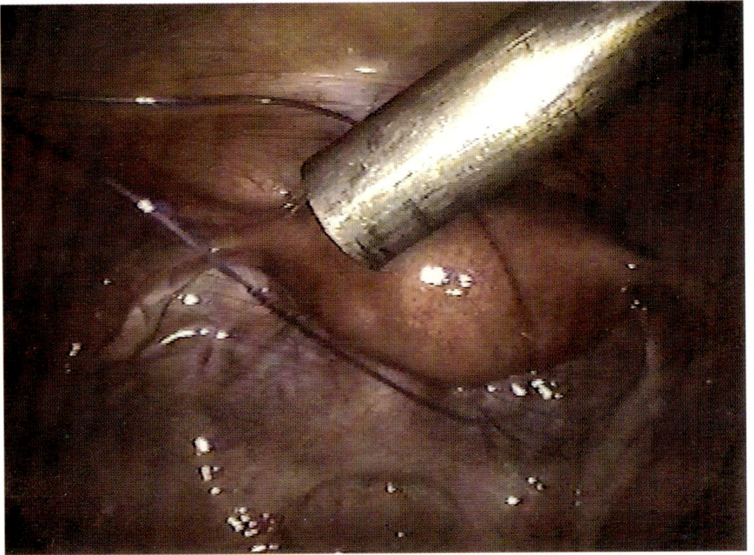

**49**

- The loop is opened with the grasping forceps
- The appendix is grasped and pulled into the loop

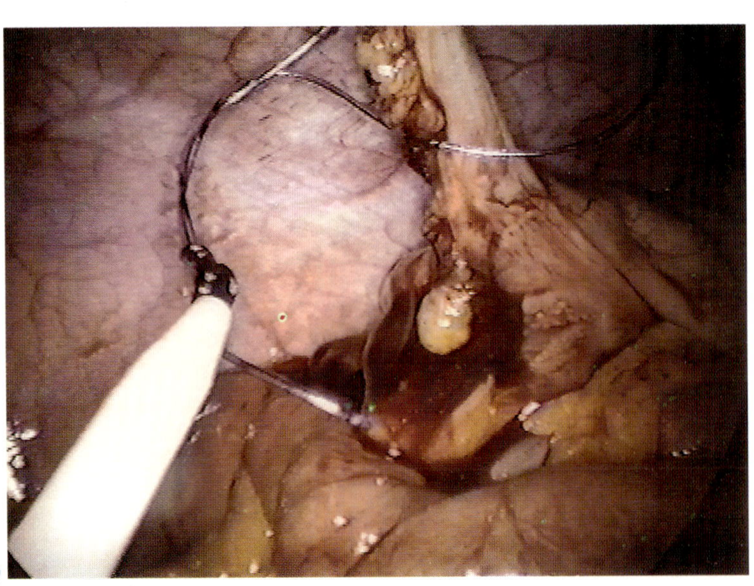

**50**

- The loop is placed at the base of the appendix, and this is ligated

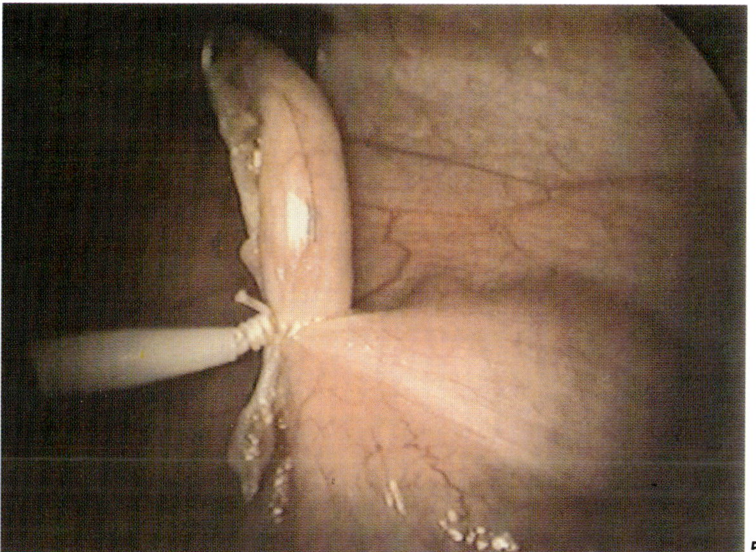

– After extraction of the knot pusher,
  the scissors are inserted parallel to
  the threads, which are cut some
  8–10 mm beyond the knot

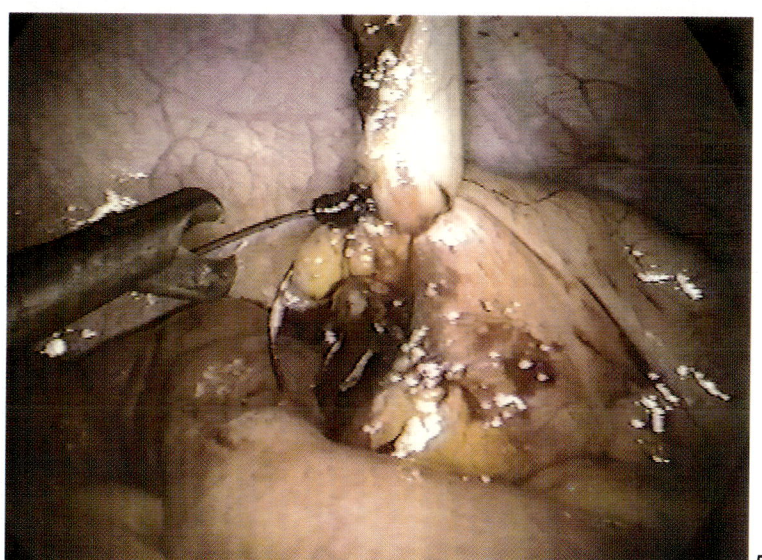

– Coagulation of the base of the appendix with bipolar high-frequency
  current (safe distance 0.5–0.7 cm)
  above the ligature

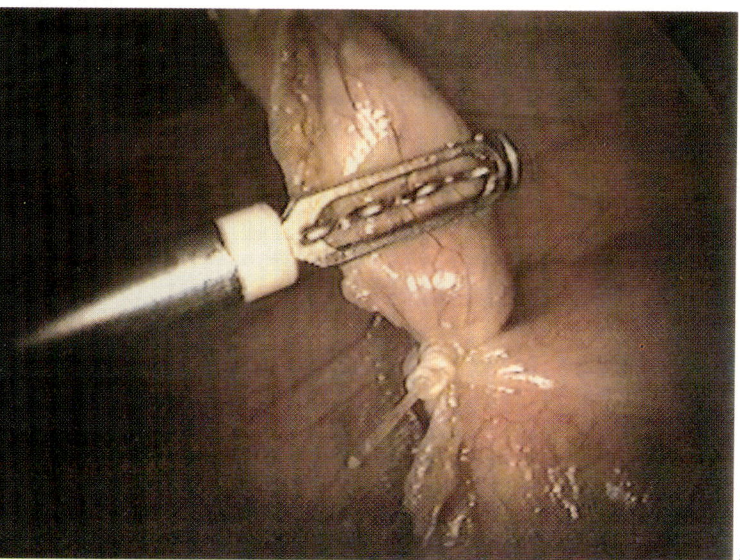

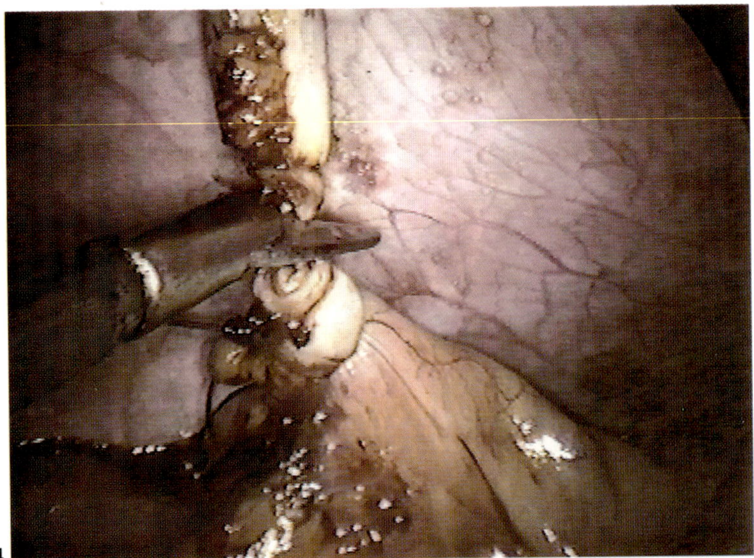

– The appendix is divided and extracted with the appendix extractor
– A phlegmonous or club-shaped, distended appendix may be removed after dilation of the incision site and replacement of the 11-mm trocar by a 15–20-mm trocar

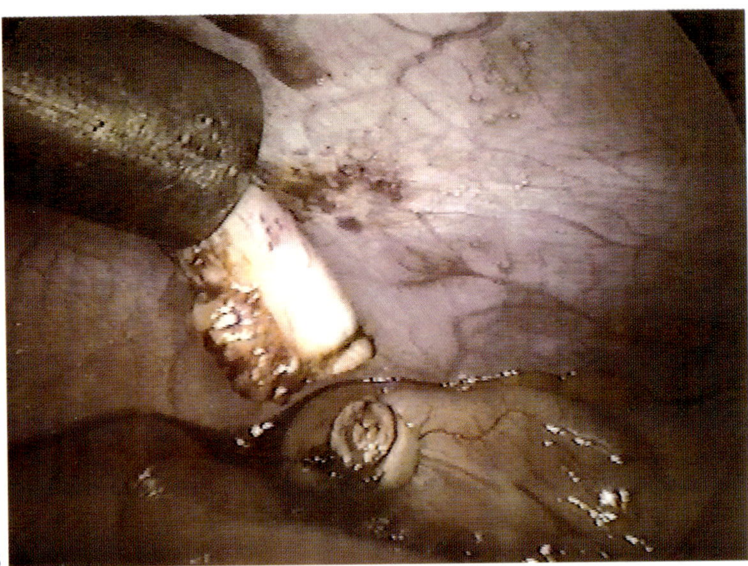

**54**

**55**

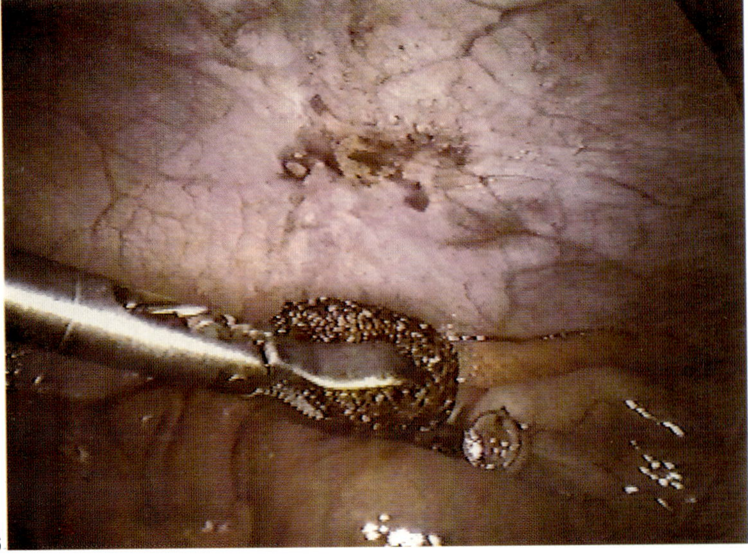

– Introduction of an iodine-impregnated dissecting swab through a second extractor sheath and disinfection of the appendix stump

**56**

## Conclusion of Appendectomy
(Figs. **57—59**)

- Optional search for Meckel's diverticulum

- Grasping of terminal ileum with atraumatic grasping forceps

- Stepwise exposure of the ileum in front of the laparoscope

- Aspiration of secretions from the space of Douglas after discontinuation of the head-down position

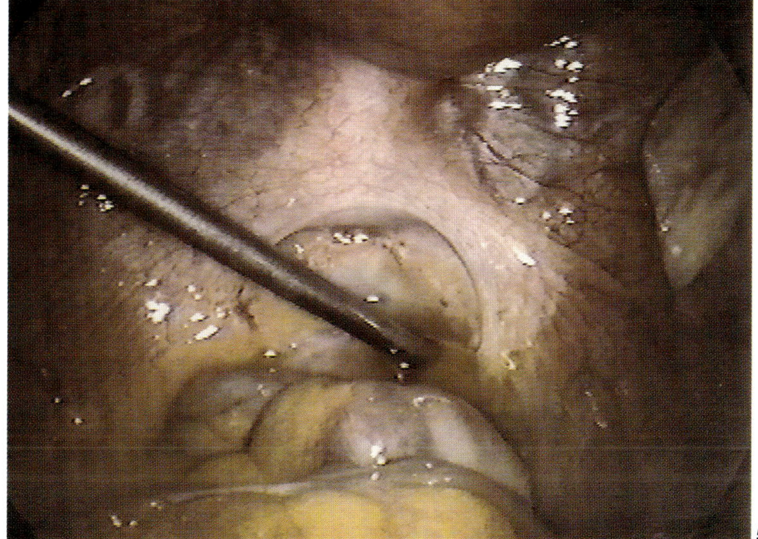

- Final inspection of the appendiceal stump

- Possibly, irrigation of the operative site

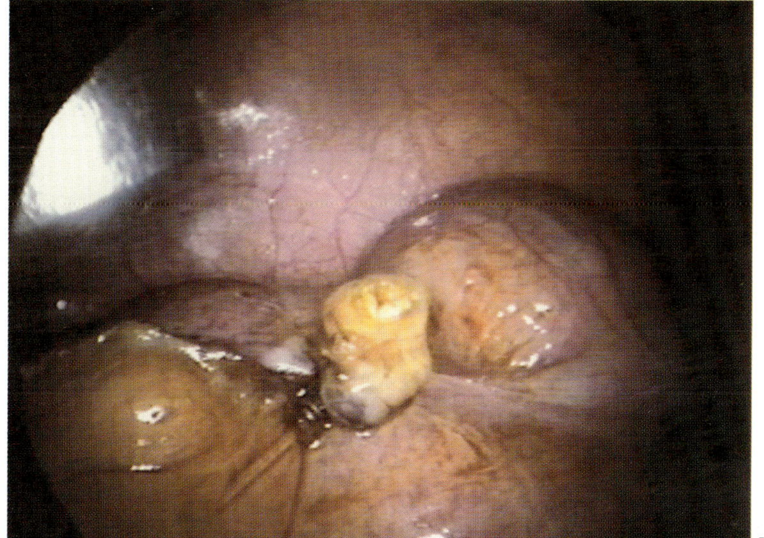

- The stump is covered with cecum or terminal ileum

- The operating trocars are withdrawn under vision *(watch out for omental tip, bleeding from puncture channel!)*

- Evacuation of pneumoperitoneum

- Suture of skin

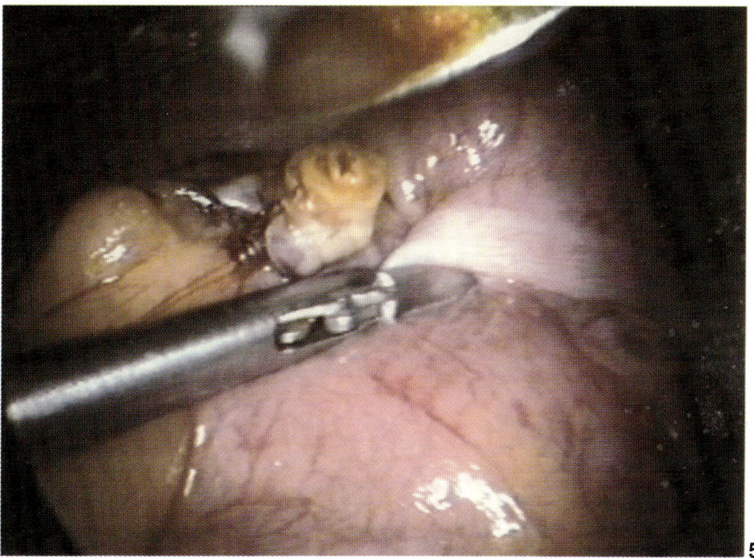

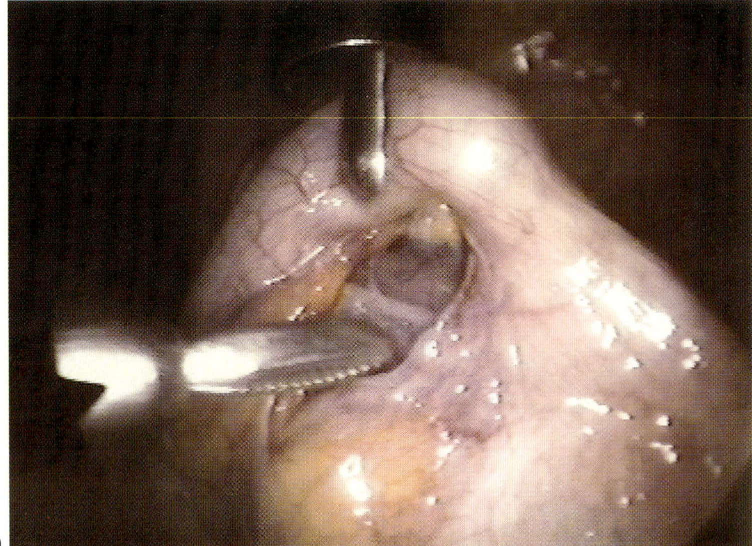

60

**Retrograde Procedure**
(Figs. **60–62**)

– The appendix is grasped near the base with the grasping forceps, and its mesentery is stretched by traction toward the abdominal wall

– The mesentery is fenestrated near the base (e.g., with scissors)

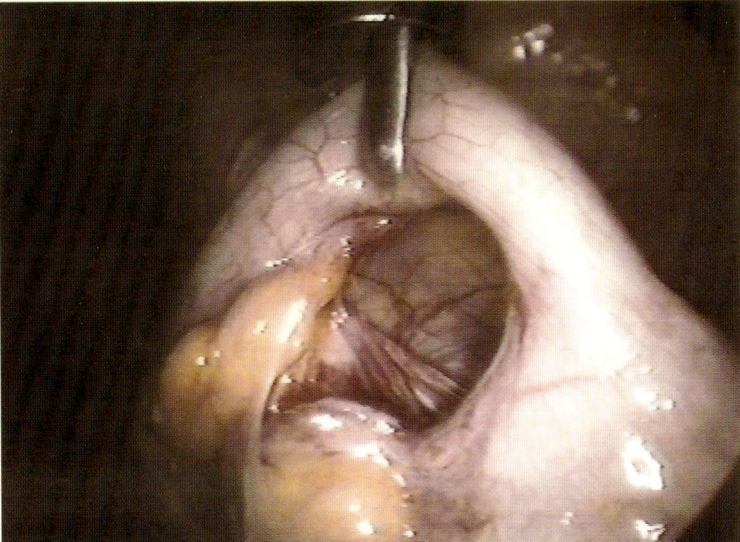

61

– The base is dissected free circularly

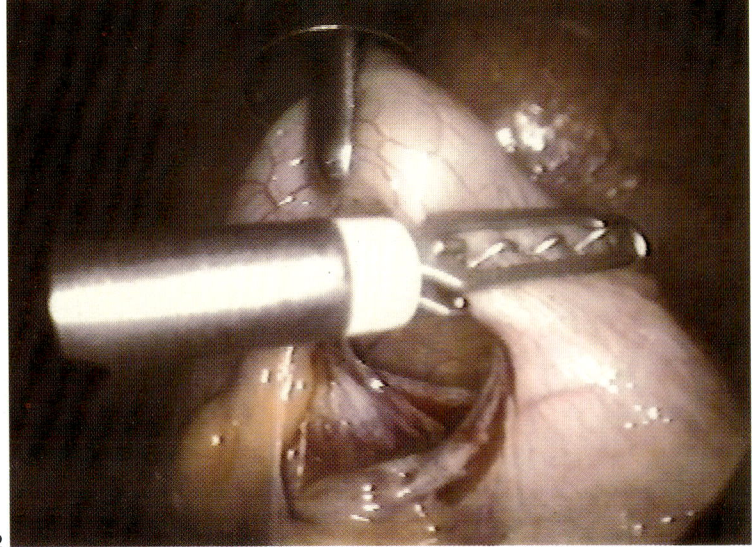

62

– Coagulation with high-frequency bipolar forceps

(Figs. **63–65**)

– The base of the appendix is transected with scissors

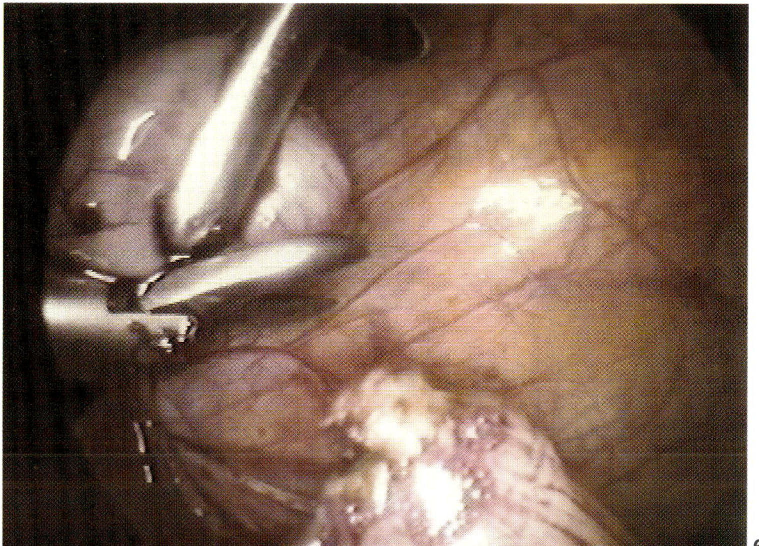

63

– The loop applicator with the Roeder loop is inserted via the 5.5-mm trocar, and the loop is placed over the appendiceal stump

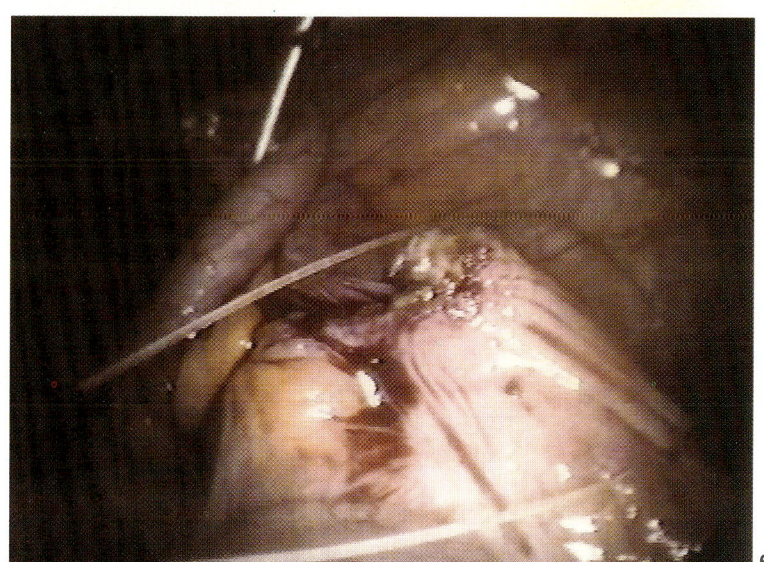

64

– The appendix stump is grasped with atraumatic grasping forceps, and the stump is pulled into the Roeder loop

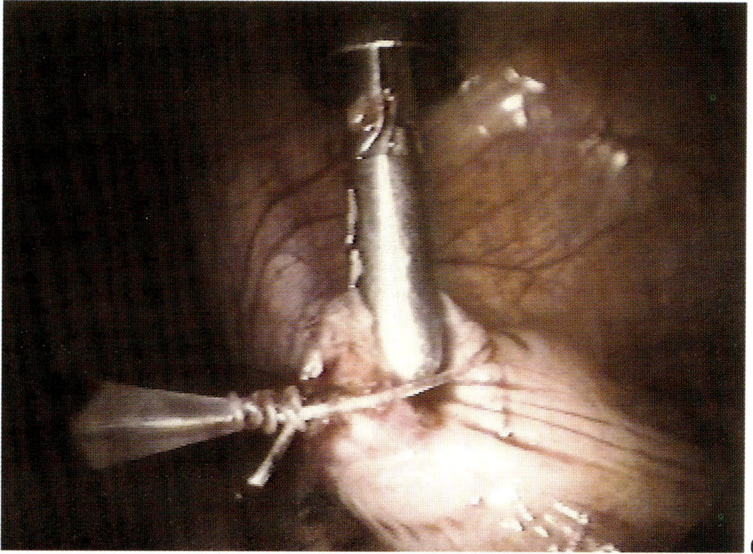

65

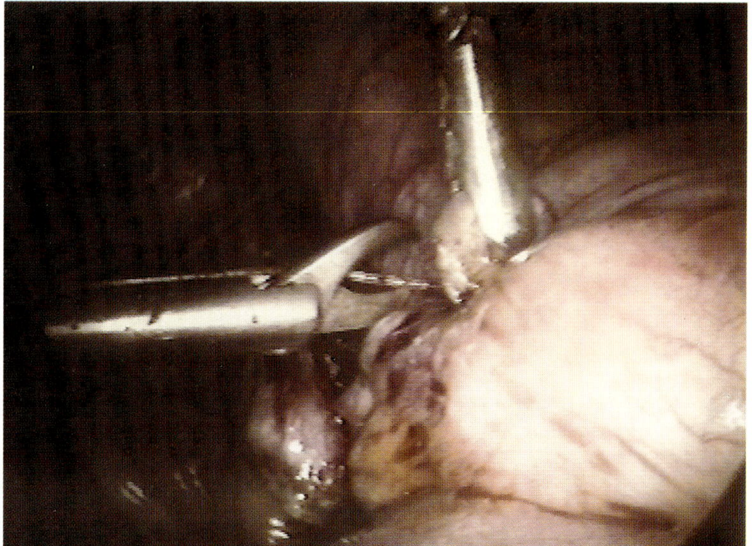

(Figs. **66–68**)

– Ligation of the stump and cutting of the suture

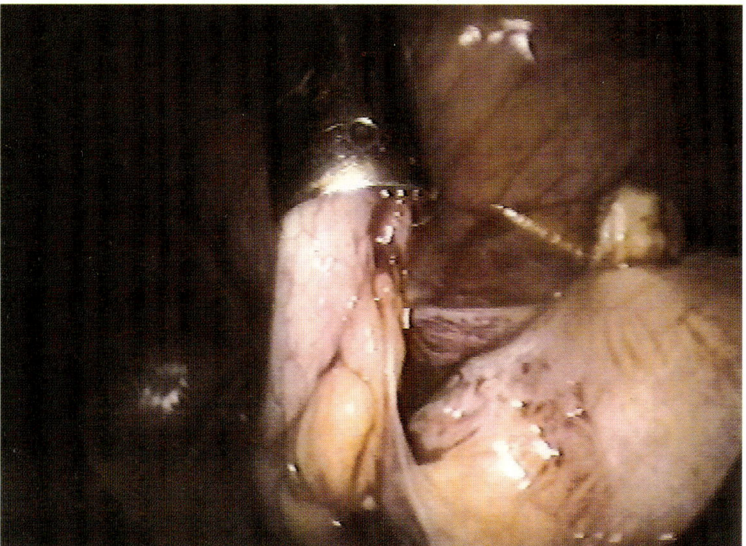

– The appendix base is grasped with atraumatic grasping forceps and pulled into the extractor sheath

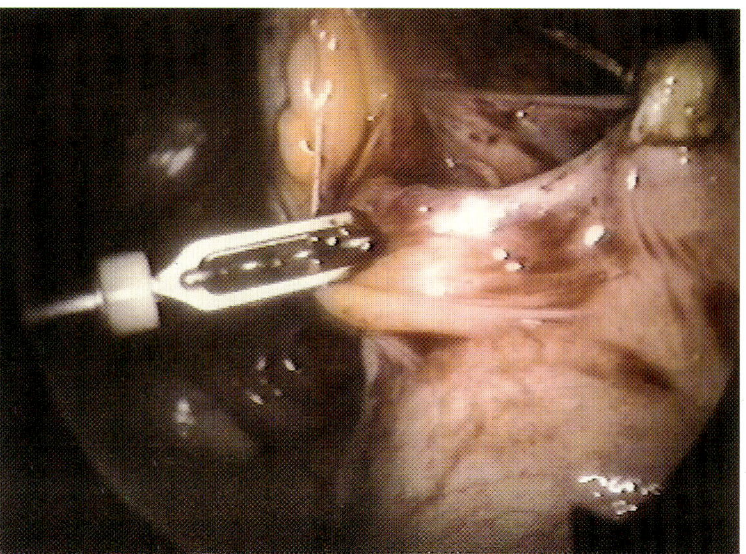

– Stepwise skeletization of the appendix coagulation of the mesentery and division as in the anterograde procedure

– Extraction of appendix

## Ruptured Appendix
(Figs. **69—71**)

- See also the chapter on Indications
- Aspiration of secretions from the space of Douglas and right lower abdomen
- Search for base of appendix with palpation probe

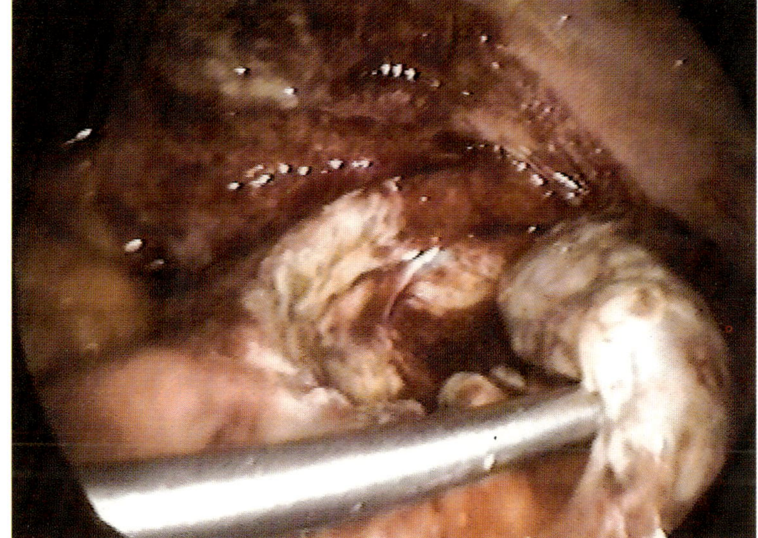

69

- Localization of perforation site
- If the perforation is near the base, conversion to laparotomy is indicated for secure closure of the stump
- If the perforation is far from the base, the appendix is circularly dissected free at the base
- The appendix is coagulated with the high-frequency bipolar forceps and divided
- The stump is grasped and retracted into the Roeder loop as in the anterograde procedure
- Stepwise anterograde or retrograde dissection of the appendix from its surroundings, depending on the position

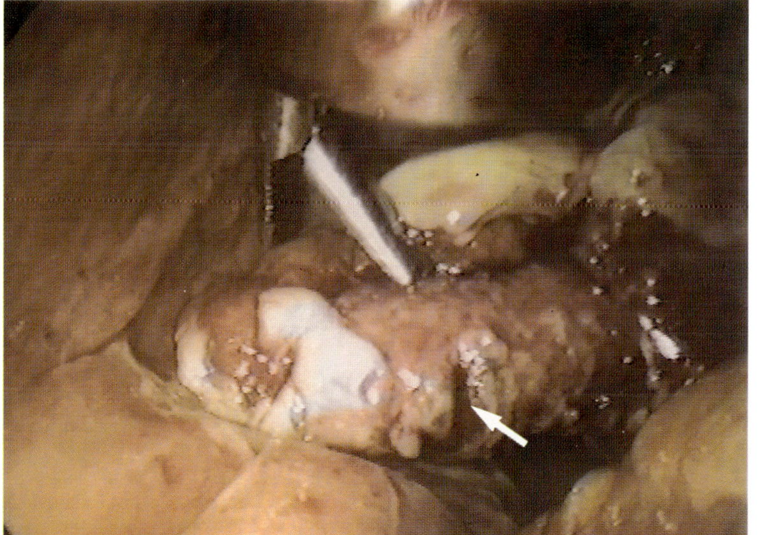

70

- Irrigation of the wound site and aspiration of secretions
- Insertion of a 5-mm silicone drain via the extractor sheath with the 11-mm trocar
- The tip is grasped and placed in the wound area
- The trocars are withdrawn under vision *(watch out for dislocation of the drain!)*

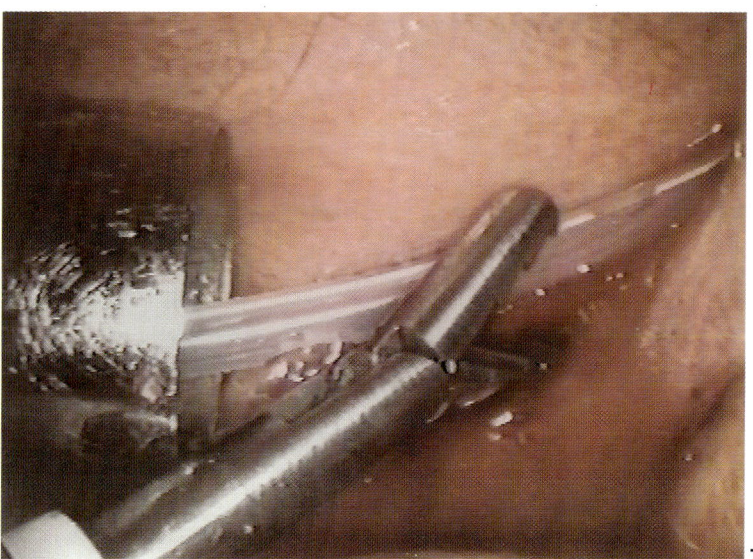

71

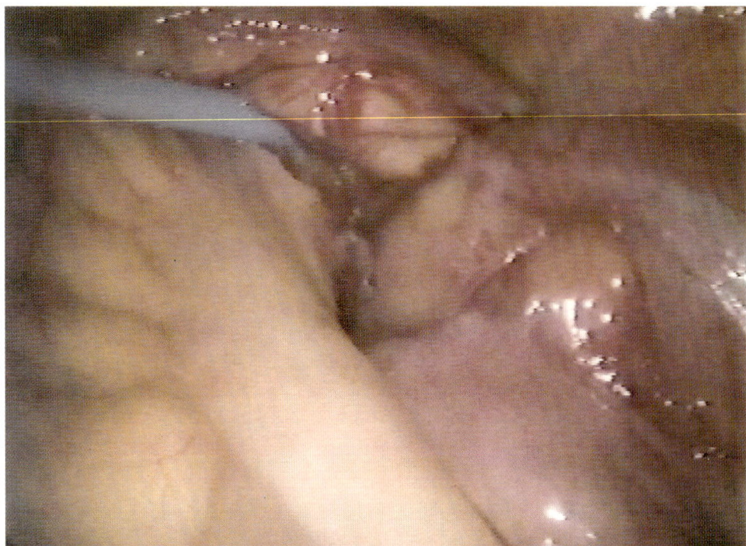

72

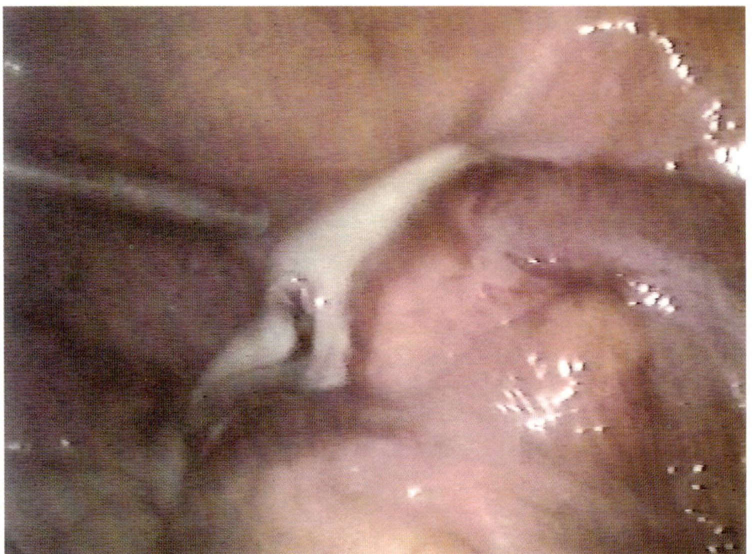

73

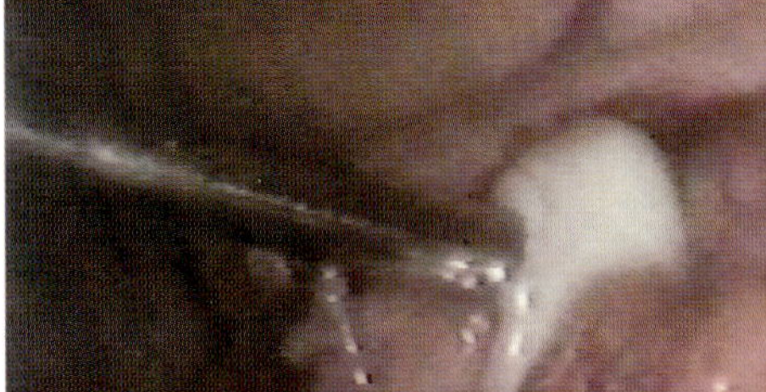
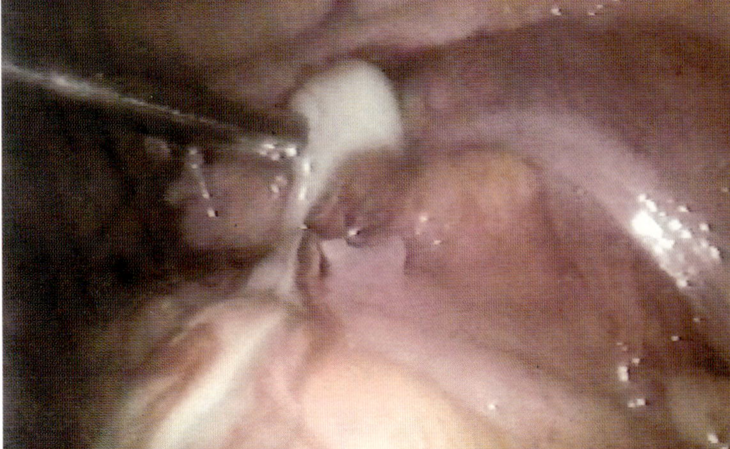

74

## Perityphlitic Abscess
(Figs. **72—74**)

- See also the chapter on Indications
- Blunt or sharp opening of the abscess membrane

- Aspiration of secretions and collection of a smear and culture
- Irrigation of abscess cavity
- The appendix is left in place
- Insertion of a 5-mm silicone drain in the extractor sheath using the 11-mm trocar
- This is grasped with the atraumatic forceps and placed in the abscess cavity
- The trocars are withdrawn under vision *(watch for dislocation of the drain!)*

# Cholecystectomy

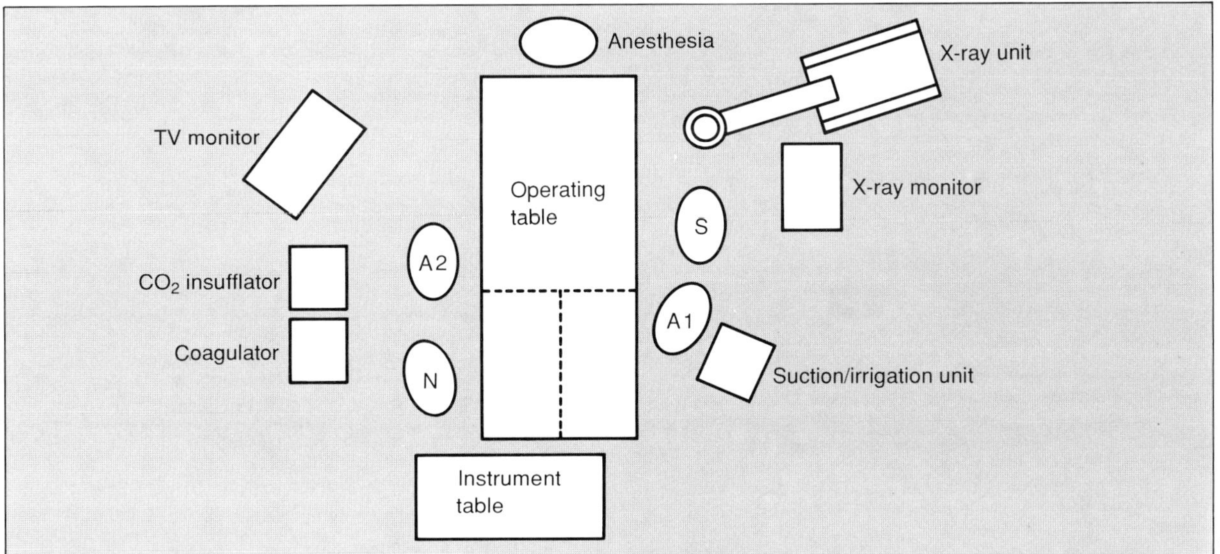


## Disposition of Equipment and Position of Surgical Team
(Fig. **75**)

- The surgeon (S) and the first assistant (A1) stand
  to the left of the patient
- The second assistant (A2) and the surgical nurse
  (N) are to the right of the patient
- The monitor and the $CO_2$ insufflator are to be
  placed in the line of vision of the surgeon and the
  first assistant
- The camera is operated by the first assistant
- Irrigation and suction are placed separately from
  the light source and the $CO_2$ insufflator
- Instrument table at the foot

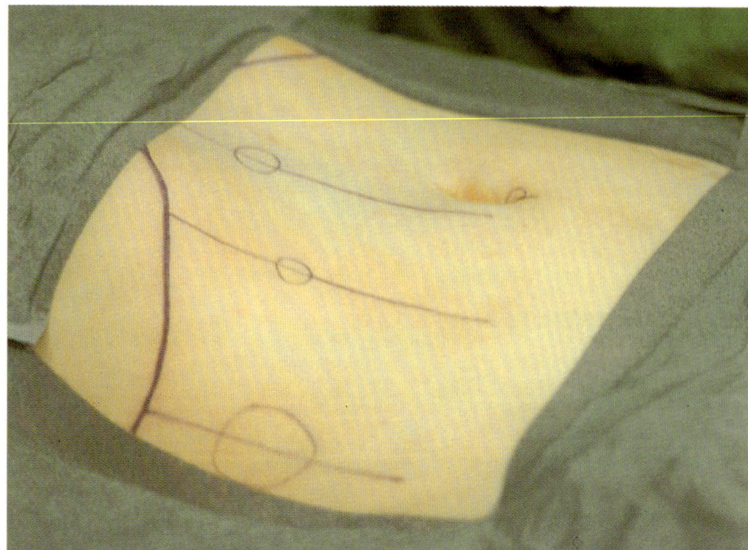

76

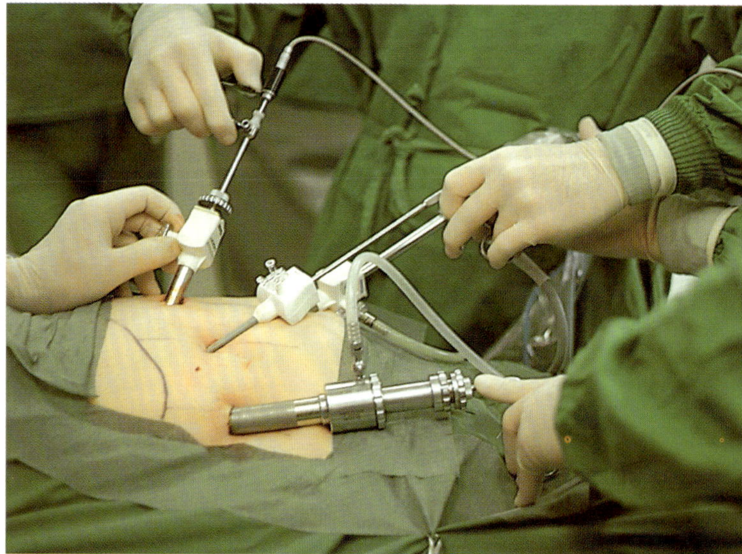

77

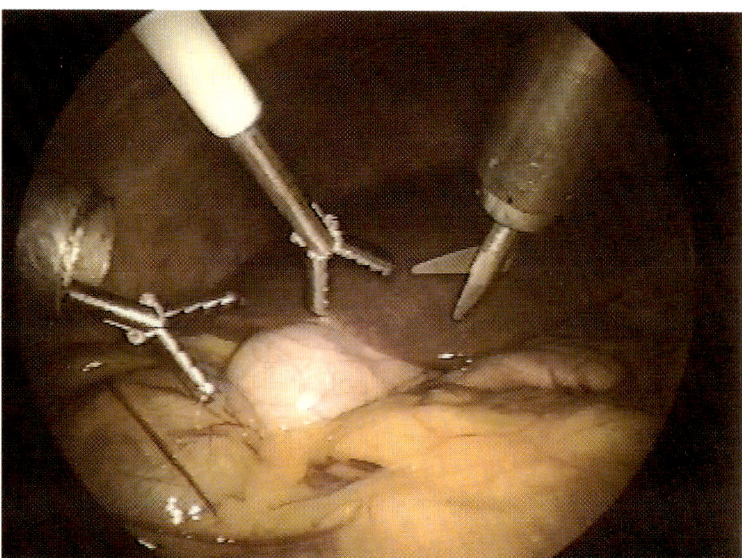

78

## Approaches into the Abdominal Cavity
(Figs. 76–78)

- Arcuate incision at the superior border of the umbilicus, 1.0–1.5 cm

- Induction of pneumoperitoneum

- Insertion of an 11-mm trocar for the forward-viewing laparoscope

- Diagnostic panoramic inspection, evaluation of operability

- Reverse Trendelenburg (10°–20°) and left lateral positioning (10°–20°)

- Three additional operating trocars are placed under endoscopic vision beneath the right costal arch

- An 11-mm trocar is placed in the right paramedian line at one-third the distance from the tip of the xiphoid and two-thirds from the umbilicus, for the dissecting instruments, scissors, suction/irrigation tube, and clip applicator *(watch out for the teres hepatis ligament!)*

- A 5.5-mm trocar is placed in the midclavicular line about 2 fingerbreadths below the costal arch, for a grasping forceps *(watch out for epigastric vessels!)*

- A 5.5-mm trocar is placed in the anterior axillary line about 3–4 fingerbreadths below the costal arch for the second grasping forceps: Optionally, a trocar of 15–20 mm is substituted for subsequent extraction of the gallbladder *(watch out for the right colon flexure!)*

- An adequate distance of these ports from the gallbladder and between the laparoscopic and operating trocars provides for a comfortable intra-abdominal range of motion

## Exposure of the Gallbladder
(Figs. **79—82**)

– The gallbladder is grasped at the
  fundus with an atraumatic grasping
  forceps through the lateral approach

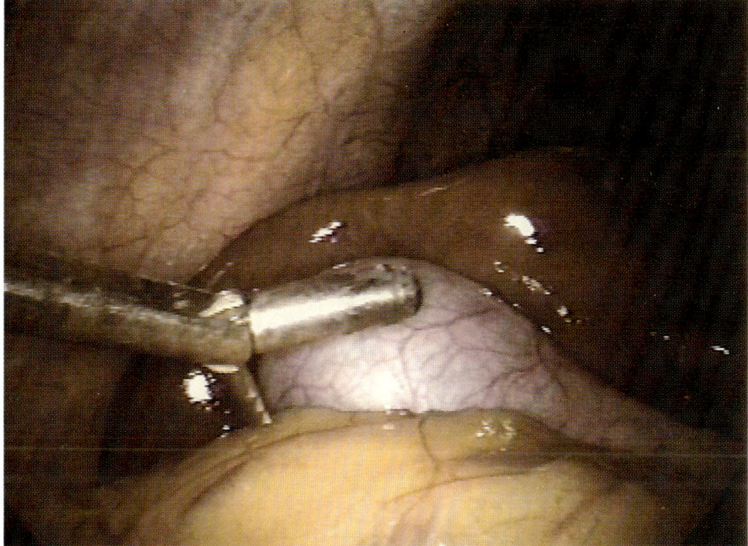

**79**

– The gallbladder and liver edge are
  elevated cranially in the direction of
  the right dome of the diaphragm by
  the assistant

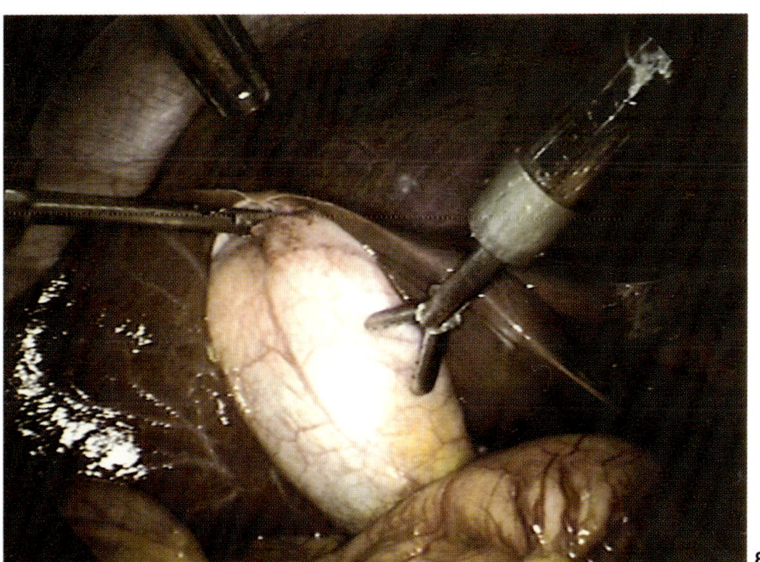

**80**

– Adhesions between the gallbladder
  and adjacent organs (omentum,
  right colon flexure, duodenum) are
  bluntly divided or transected with a
  hooked electrode or scissors

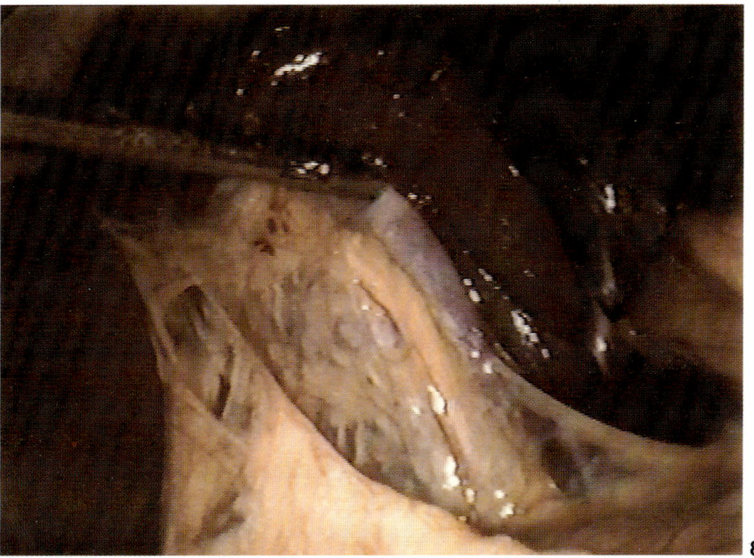

**81**

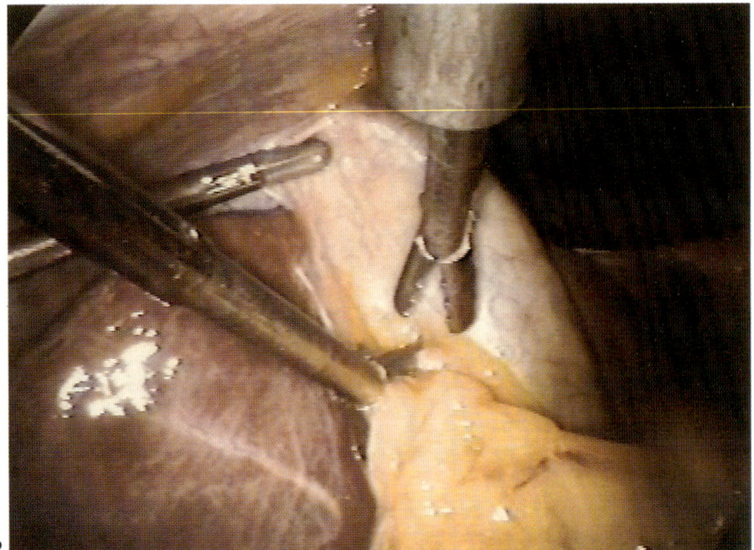

82

(Figs. **83, 84**)

- The infundibulum of the gallbladder is grasped with the second grasping forceps through the midclavicular port and retracted laterally for exposure of Calot's triangle

- Traction on or lifting of the infundibulum provides for good anterior or posterior exposure of the region

83

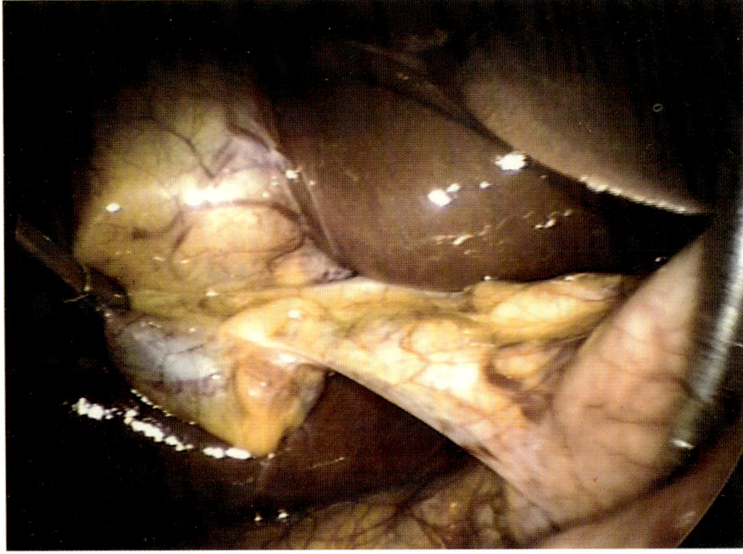

84

## Cholecystocholangiography
(Figs. **85–89**)

– The elevated gallbladder is punctured through the midclavicular approach with the DeKock grasping forceps (alternatively with a cannula penetrating through the abdominal wall)

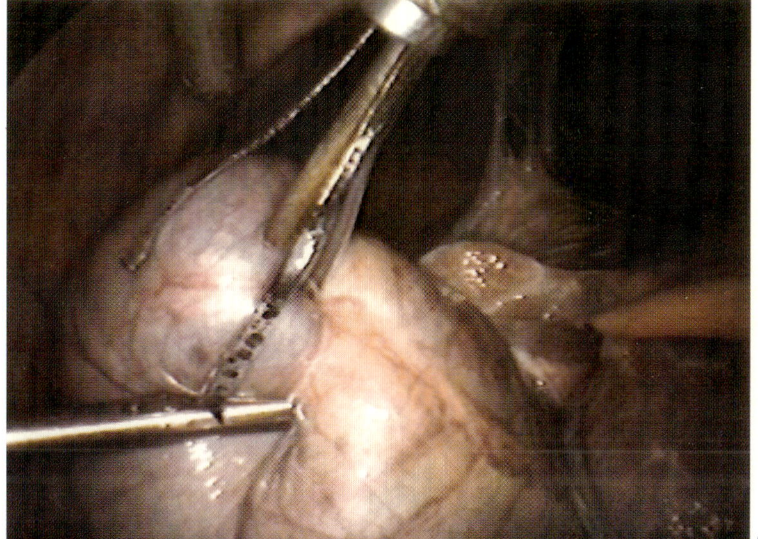

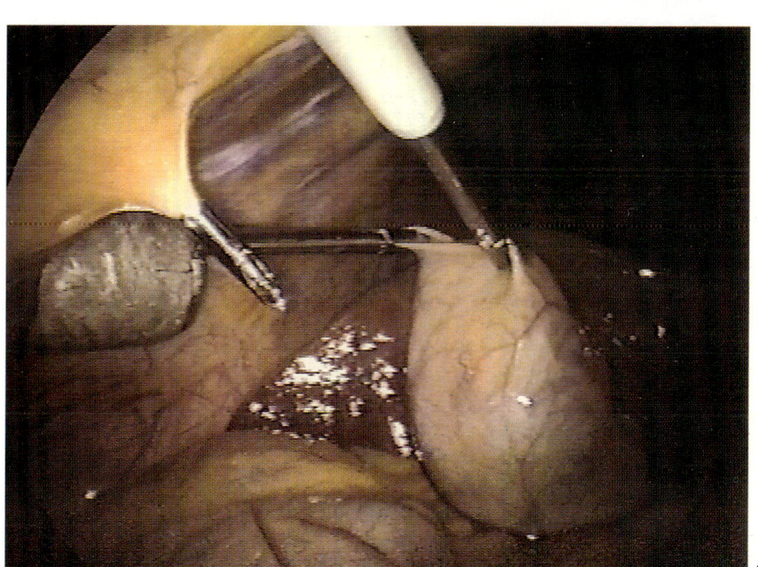

– Aspiration of bile, irrigation with saline solution, and injection of contrast material

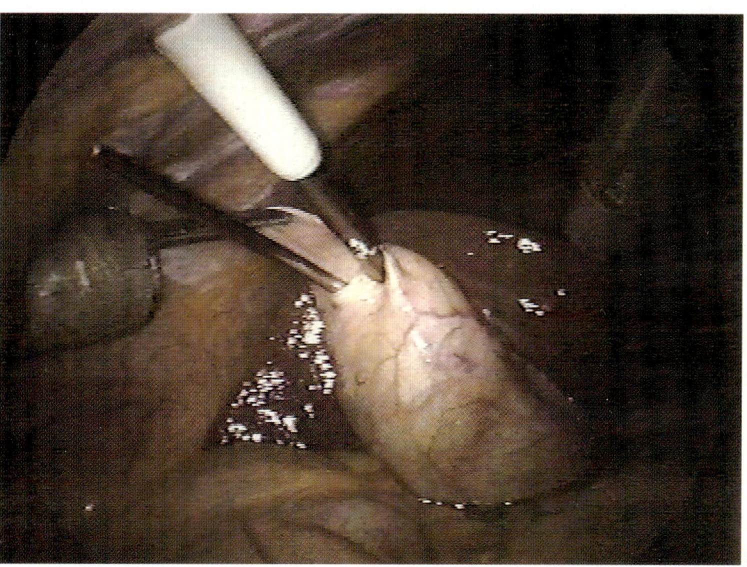

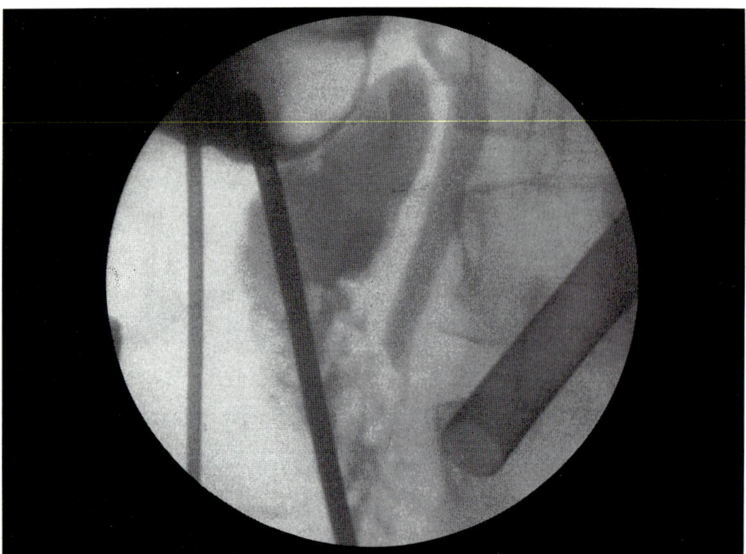

– Fluoroscopy and cholangiography of
  contrast material passing through
  the biliary tree

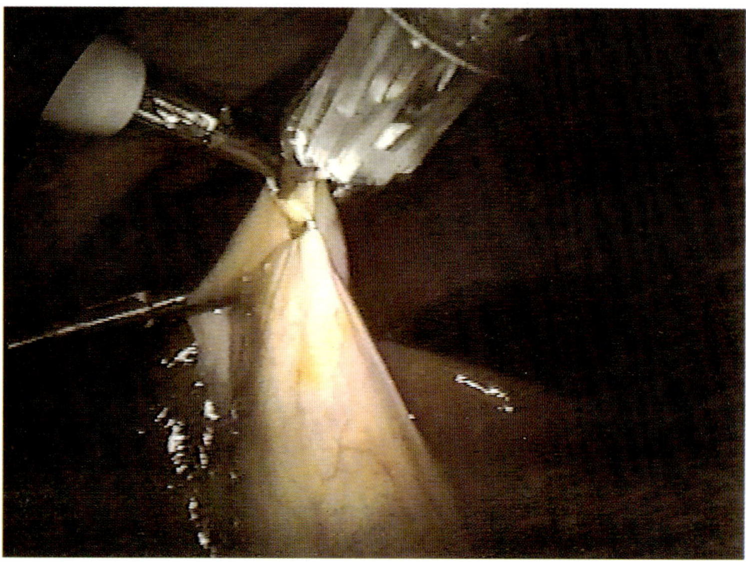

– Grasping of puncture site with lateral grasping forceps, or clip closure
  of puncture site

## Dissection of Cystic Duct and Cystic Artery
(Figs. **90—95**)

– Incision of peritoneal investment

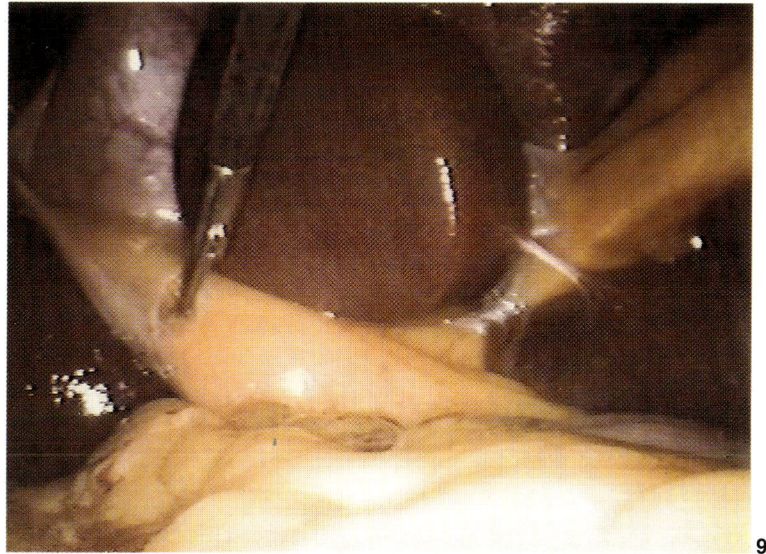

90

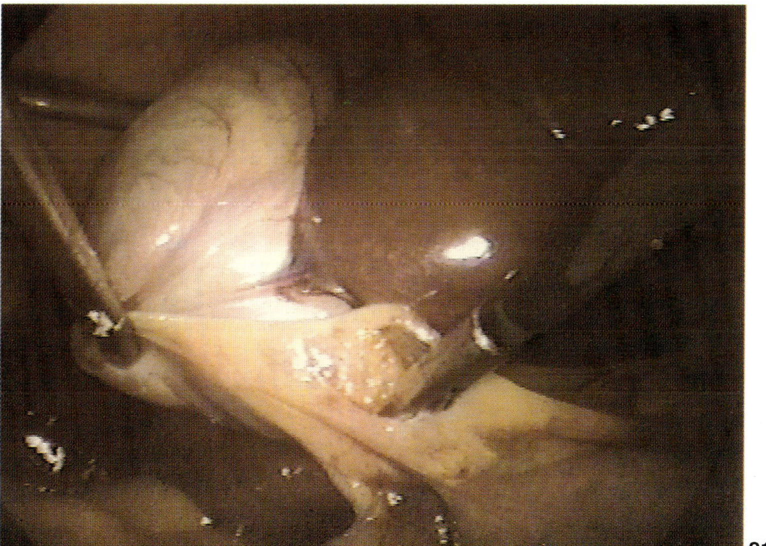

91

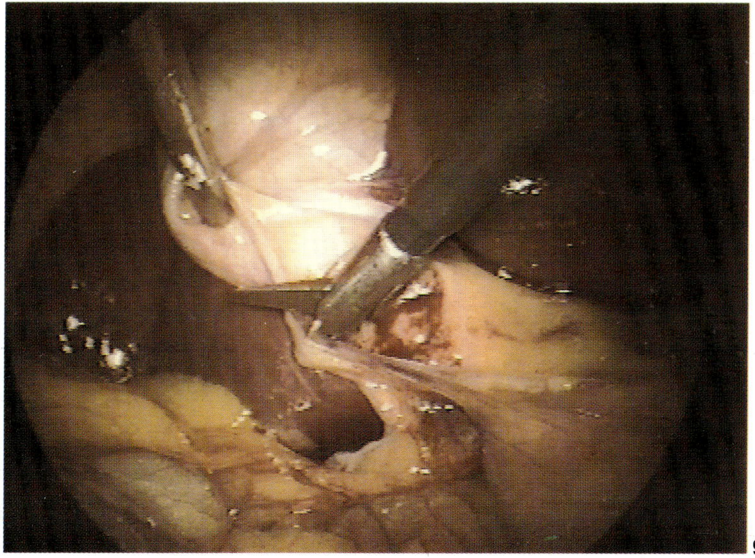

92

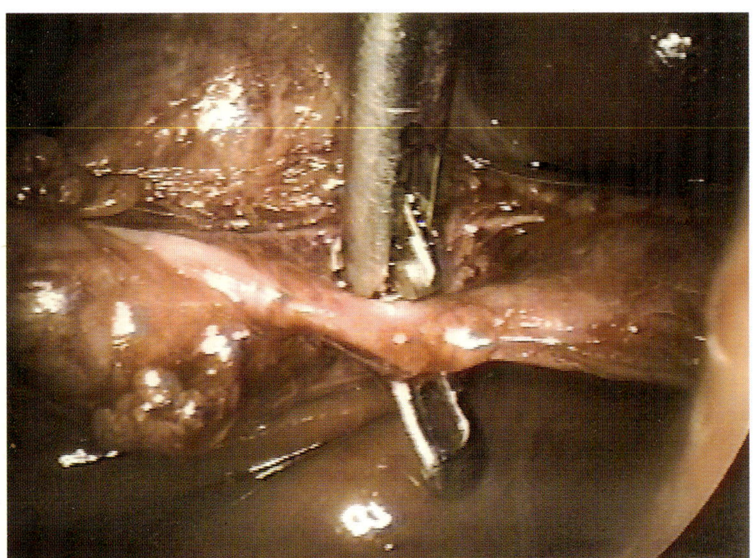

93

- The dissection is carried out with dissecting needle-nose forceps, a curved dissecting forceps, a hook electrode, or scissors
- Dissection of individual structures, begins at the infundibulum, in the direction of the common bile duct

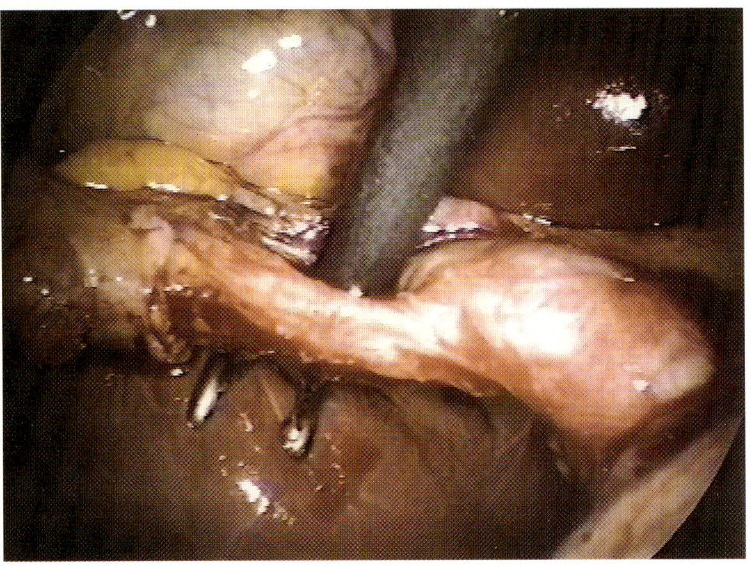

94

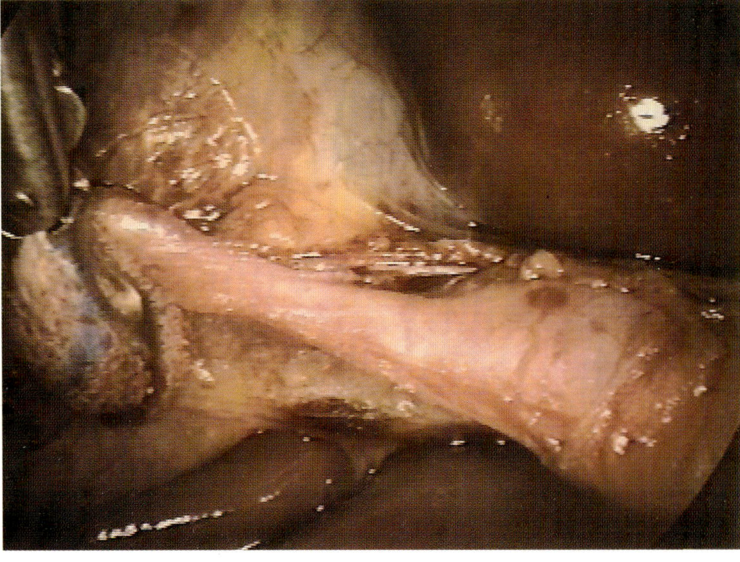

95

- Exposure of junction of the cystic duct into the hepatic duct

(Figs. **96, 97**)

– Secure application of the clips requires clear identification and complete circular exposure of the cystic
  duct and artery

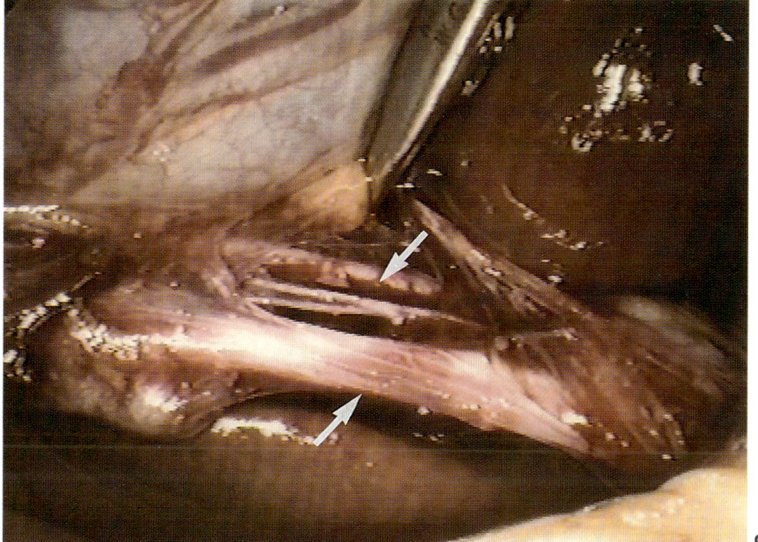

96

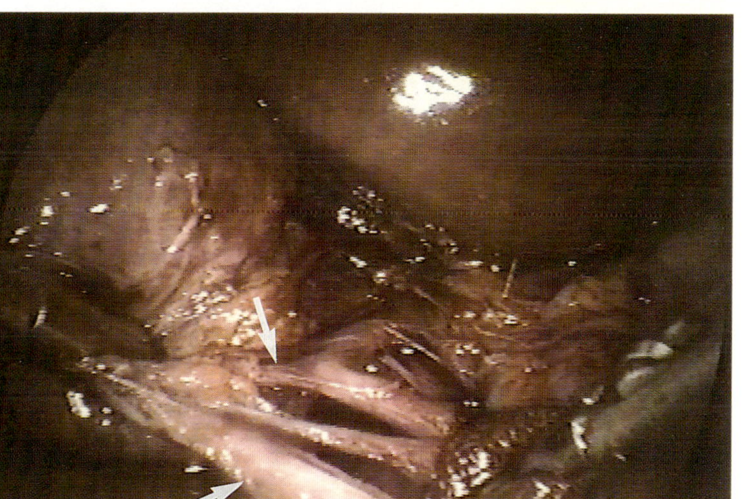

97

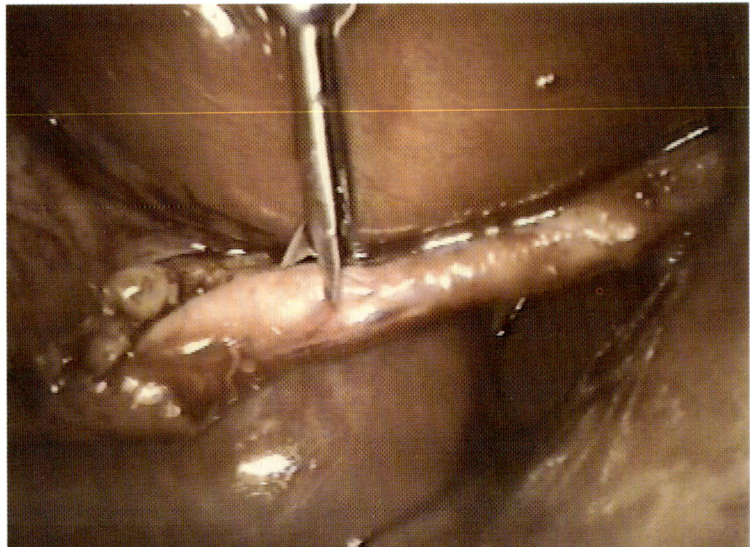

**98**

## Cholangiography
(Figs. **98–100**)

- Optional in occlusion of cystic duct by calculus

- The anterior circumference of the cystic duct is incised near the gall-bladder with microscissors

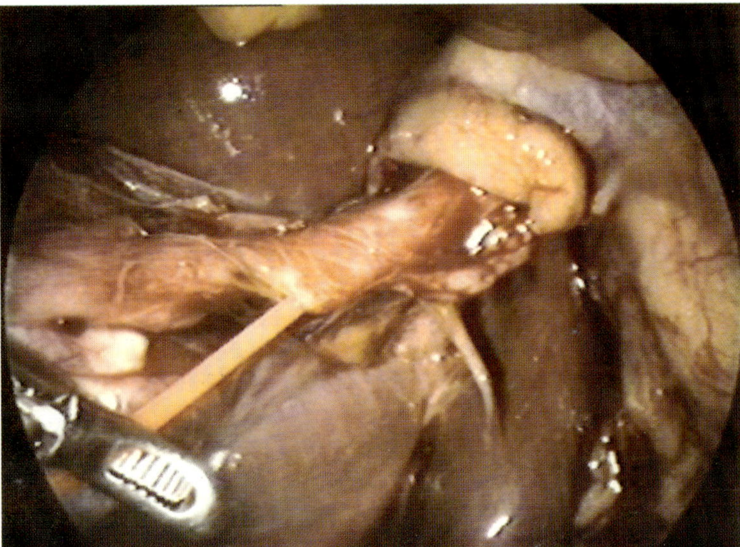

**99**

- Percutaneous passage of the balloon catheter and insertion into the cystic duct

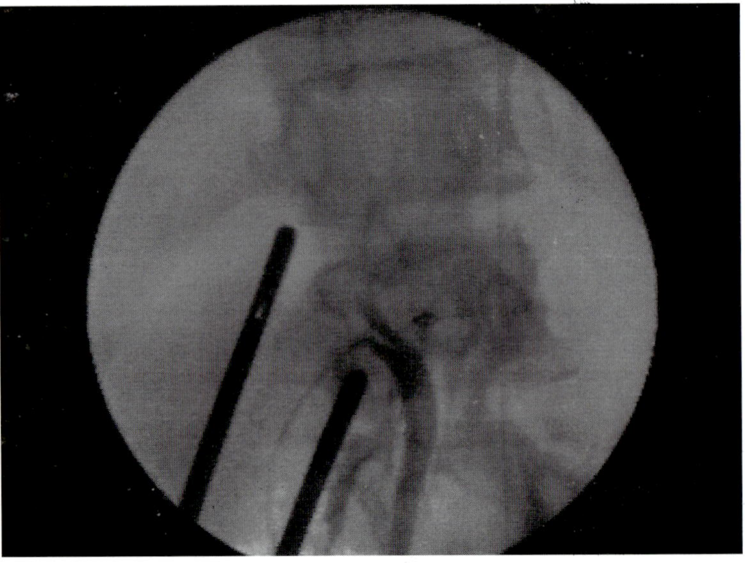

**100**

- Fluoroscopy and cholangiography

## Closure of Cystic Duct and Cystic Artery
(Figs. **101—103**)

- After circular dissection and clear identification of the cystic duct *(watch out for anatomical variations!)*

- The clip applicator (Filshie clip, titanium clip, endoclip, etc.) is inserted through the paramedian operating trocar

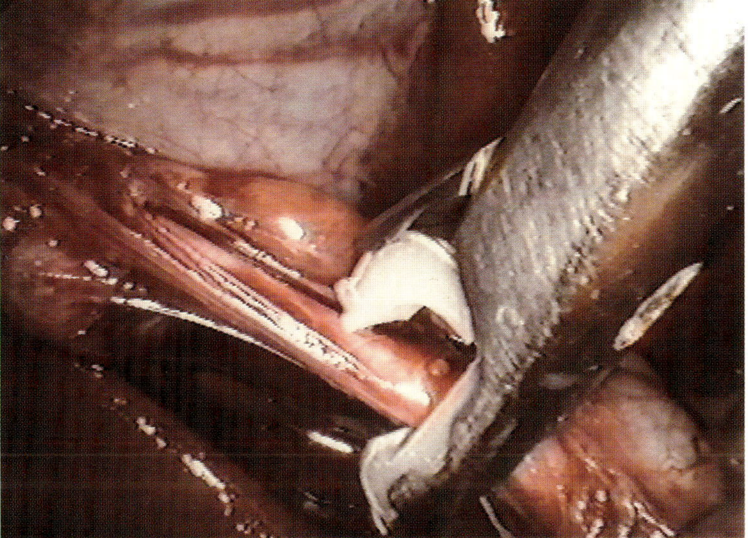

101

- The cystic duct is closed peripherally near the gallbladder and centrally near its junction with the common duct

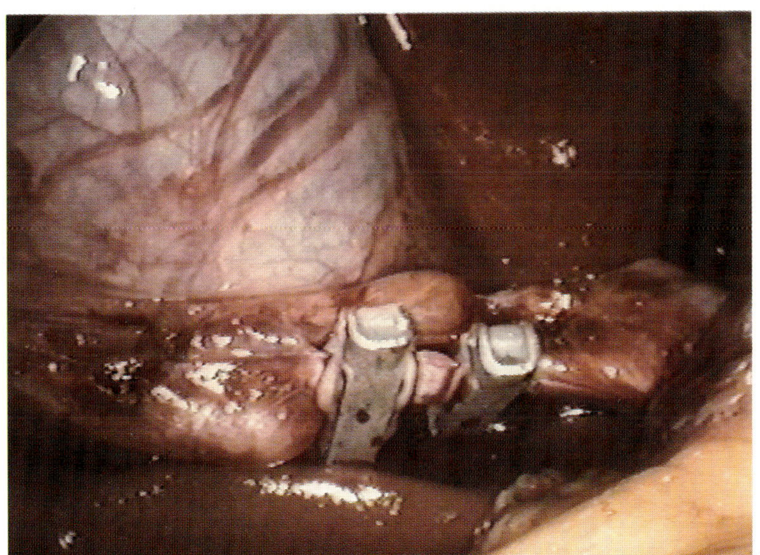

102

- Division of cystic duct between the central and peripheral clips

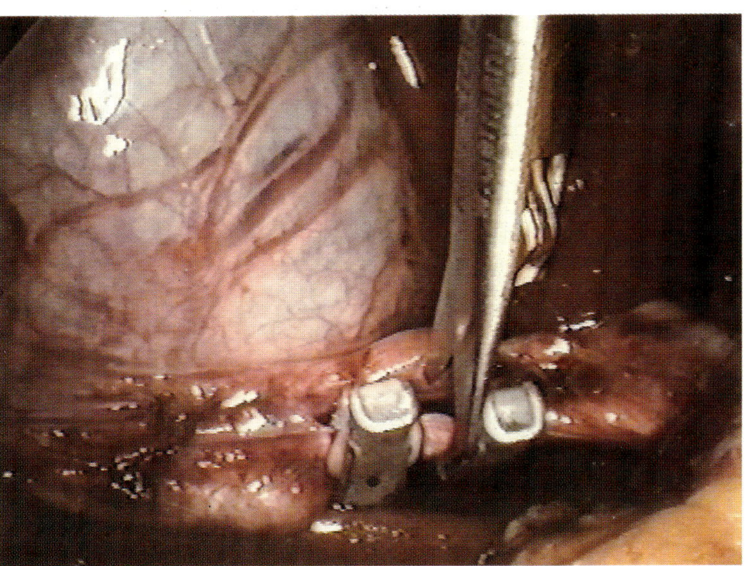

103

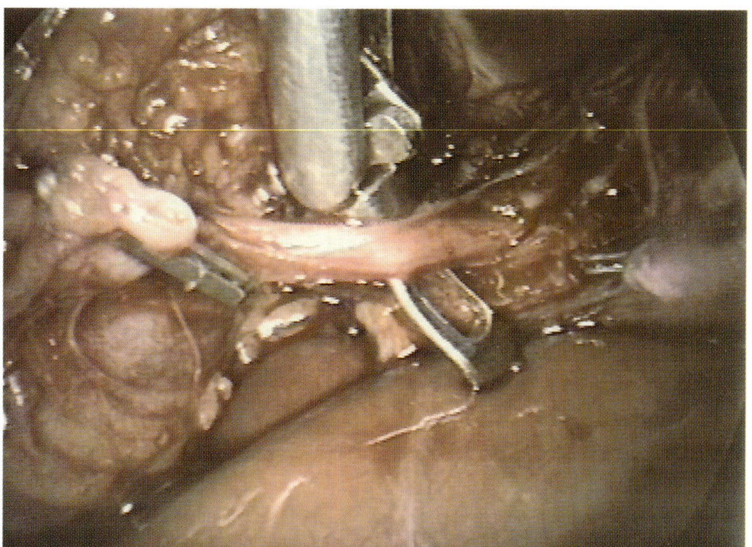

104

(Figs. **104–109**)

– Closure of the cystic duct as a first step generally permits better identification and safer closure of the cystic artery

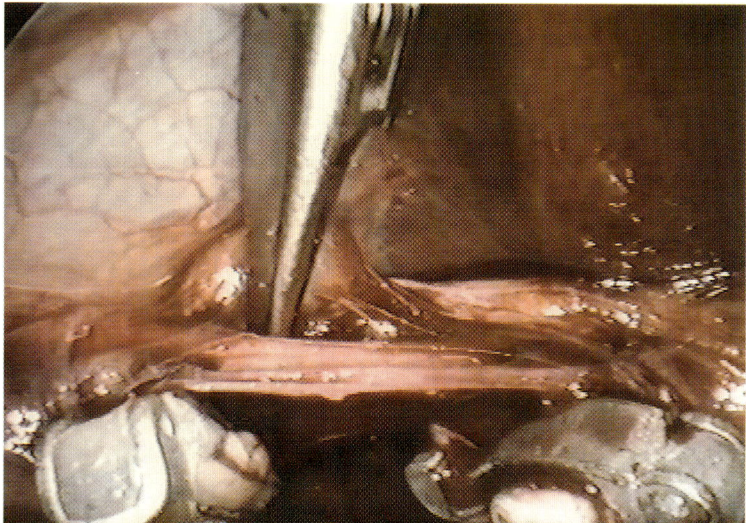

105

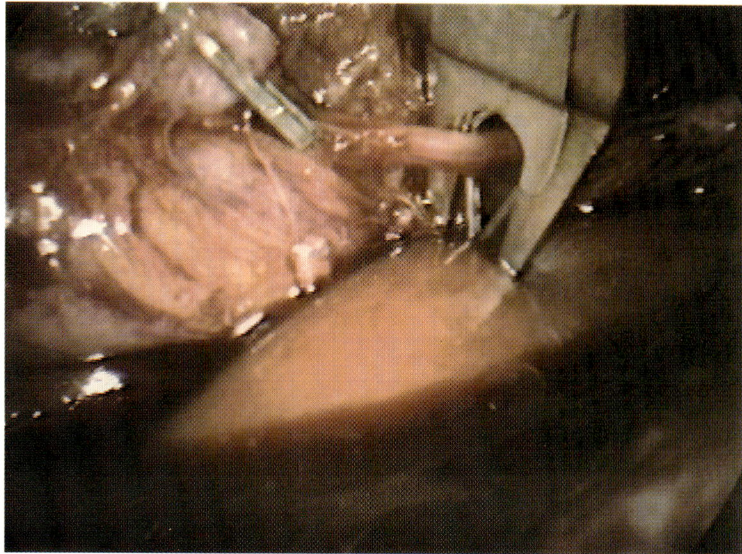

106

– Double clip ligation of the cystic artery (titanium clips or endoclip) and division with scissors between clips

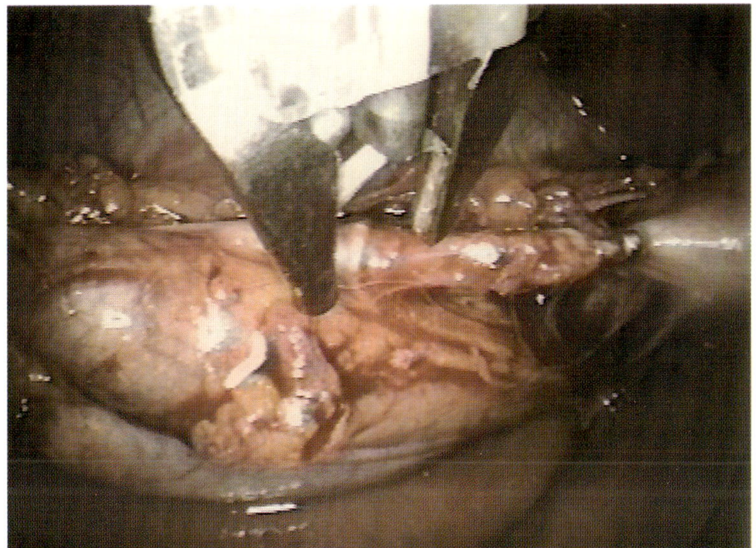

107

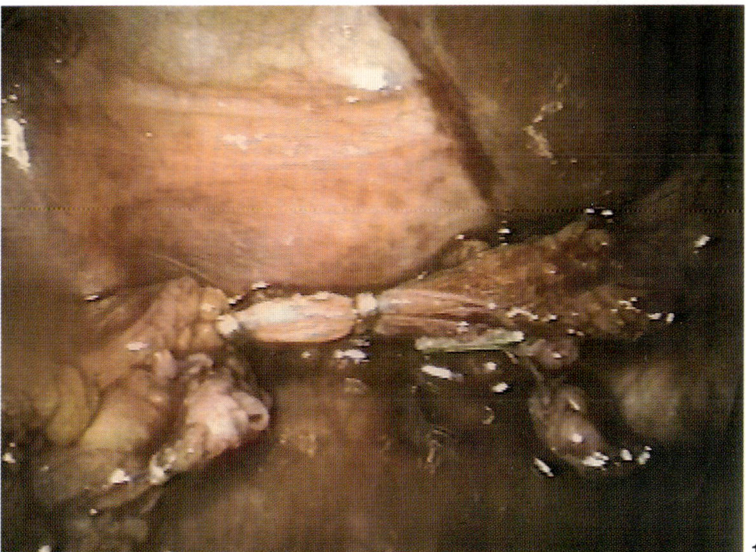

108

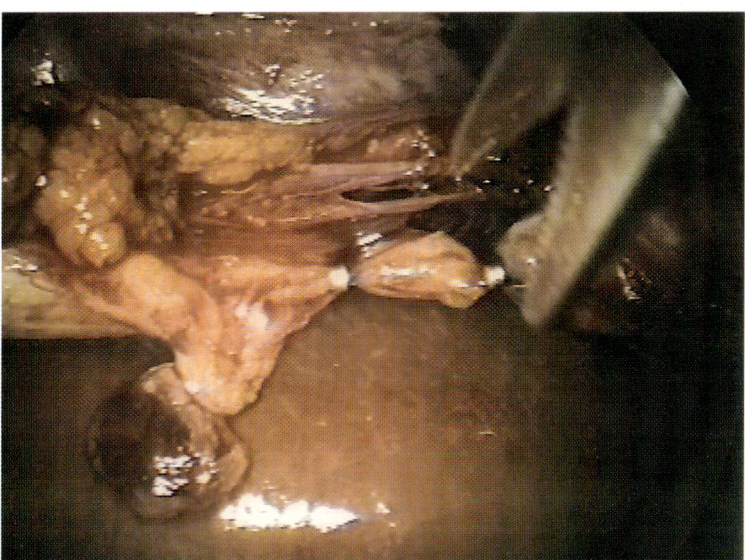

109

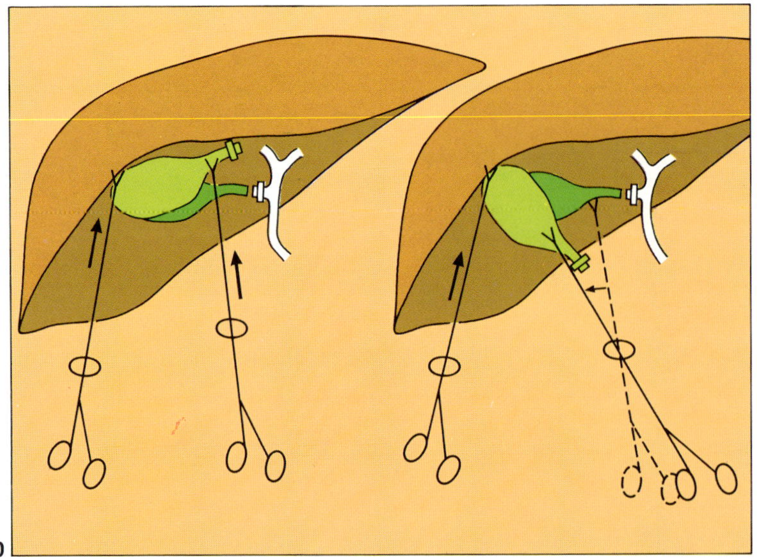

110

## Dissection of the Gallbladder
(Figs. **110—118**)

- The gallbladder is elevated by its
  fundus with a lateral grasping forceps by the assistant

- Traction on the gallbladder infundibulum with a second grasping forceps stretches the layers to be divided

- Medial superior or lateral rotation
  brings the left and right aspects of
  the gallbladder into view

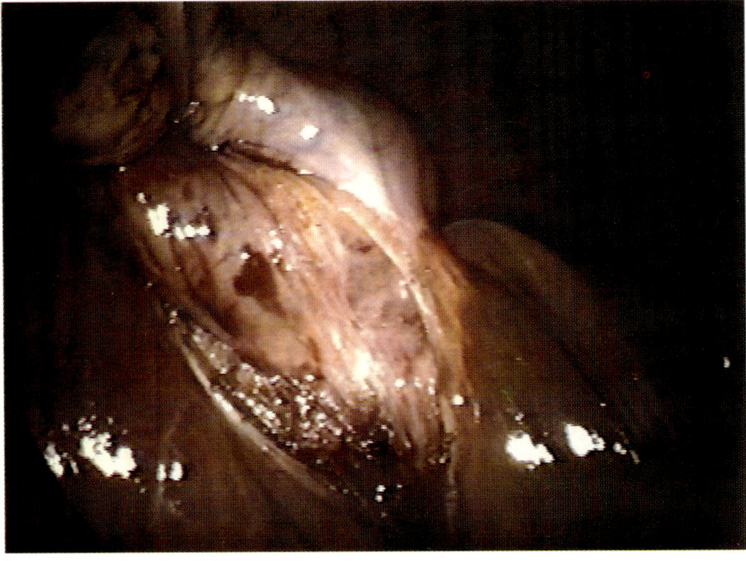

111

- The spread-out structures are separated step by step, both bluntly (dissecting forceps) and sharply (scissors), or with a hook electrode

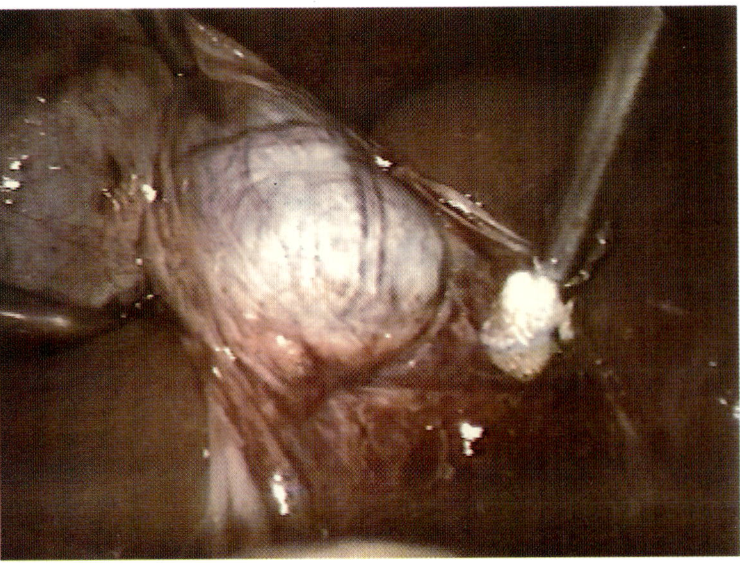

112

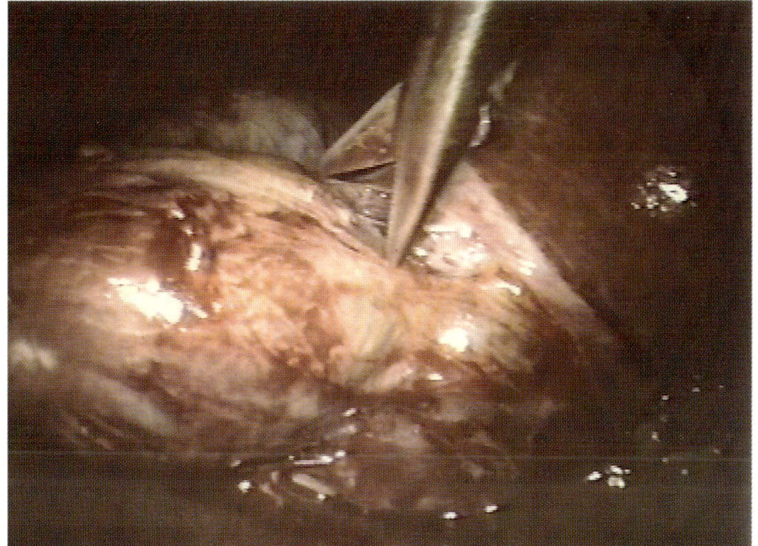

113

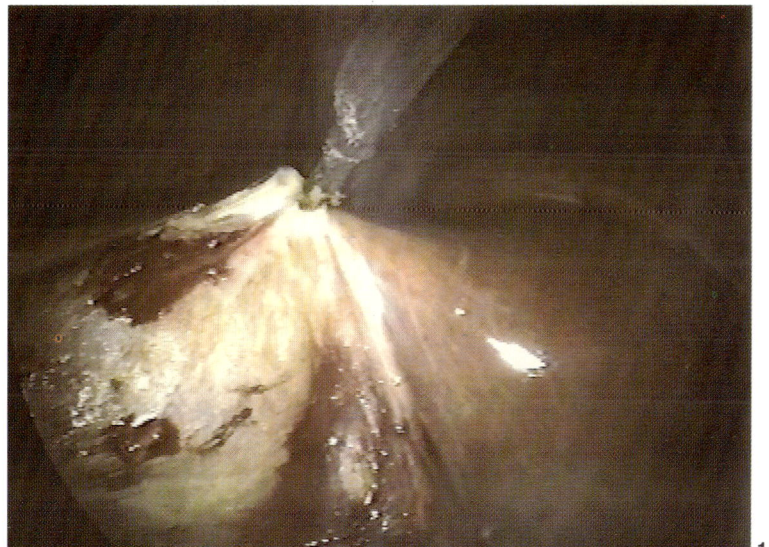

114

– Smaller, visible vessels or bleeding areas in the gallbladder bed are coagulated

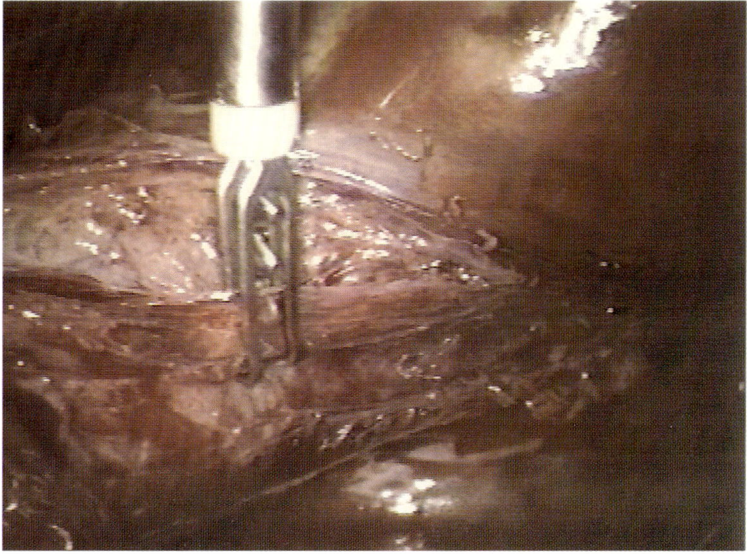

115

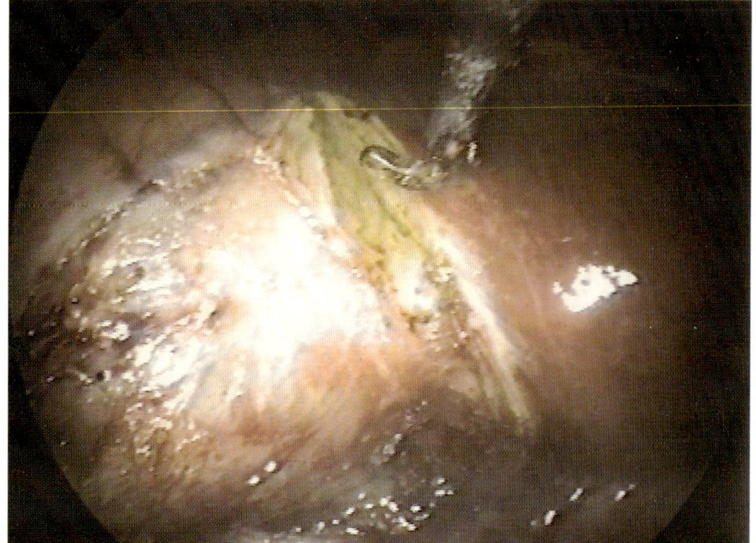

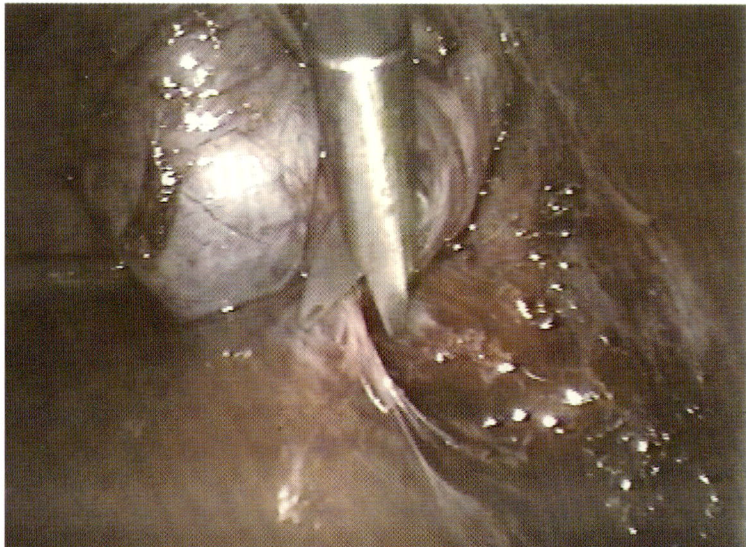

– Division of the last tissue bridges
between the gallbladder and the upper margin of the liver with the use
of scissors

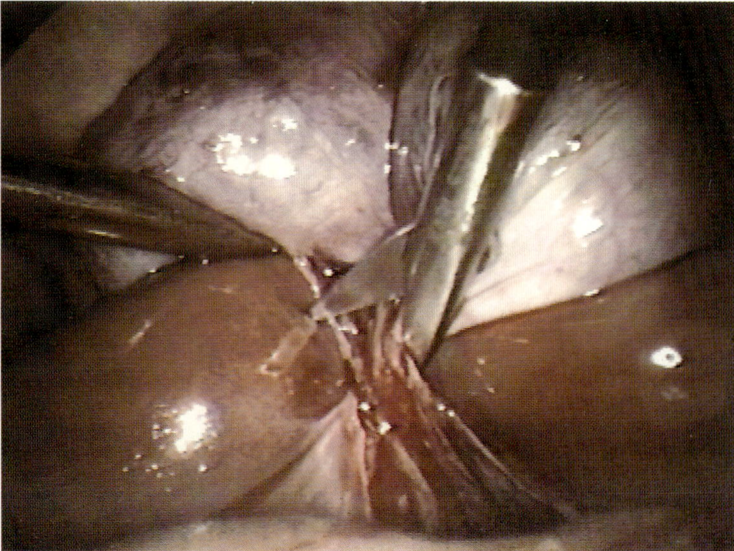

## Extraction of the Gallbladder
(Figs. **119–124**)

- This extraction is carried out via either the umbilical incision or the lateral trocar

- For extraction through the umbilical incision, the laparoscope is replaced into the paramedian 11-mm operating trocar

- For extraction through the lateral port, a 15- or 20-mm trocar sheath is required. This was either placed initially or is substituted for the 5.5-mm trocar after dilation of the 5.5-mm incision over a guide rod

- The gallbladder is grasped at the infundibulum with a heavy crocodile forceps

- It is then extracted through the abdominal wall or into the 20-mm trocar using gentle traction

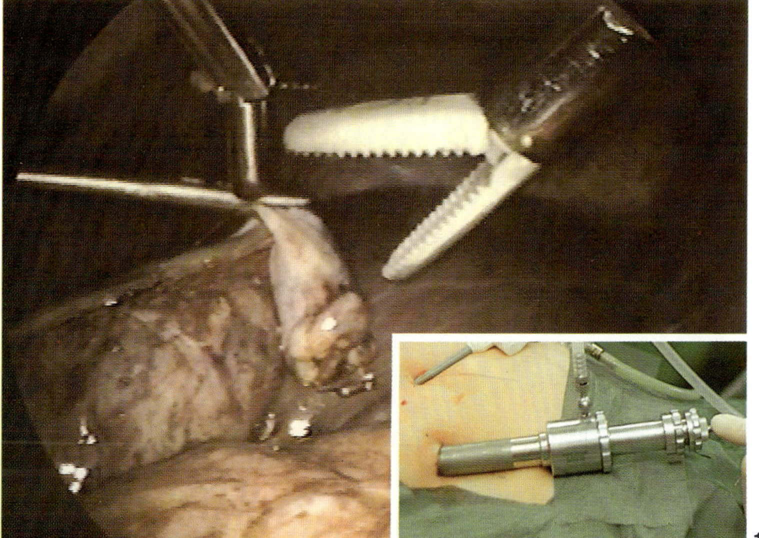

119

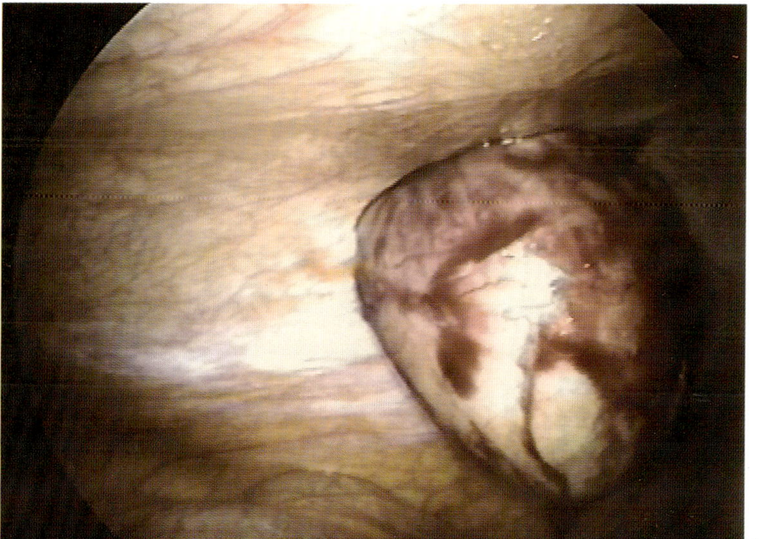

120

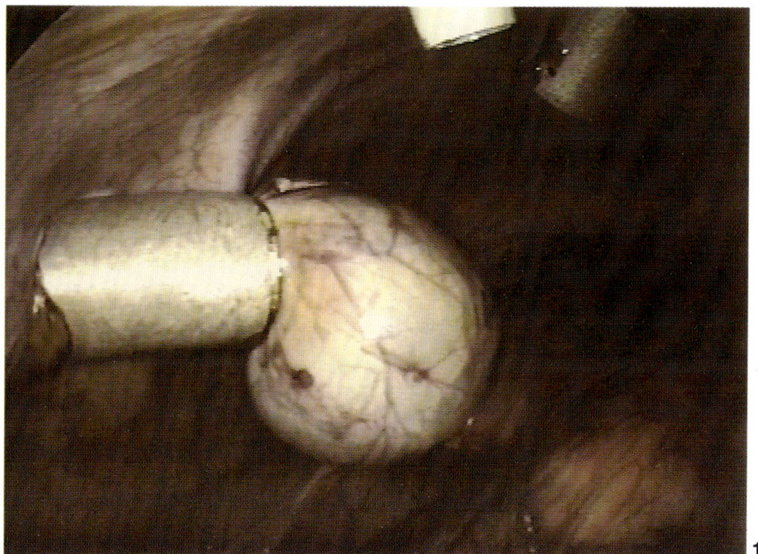

121

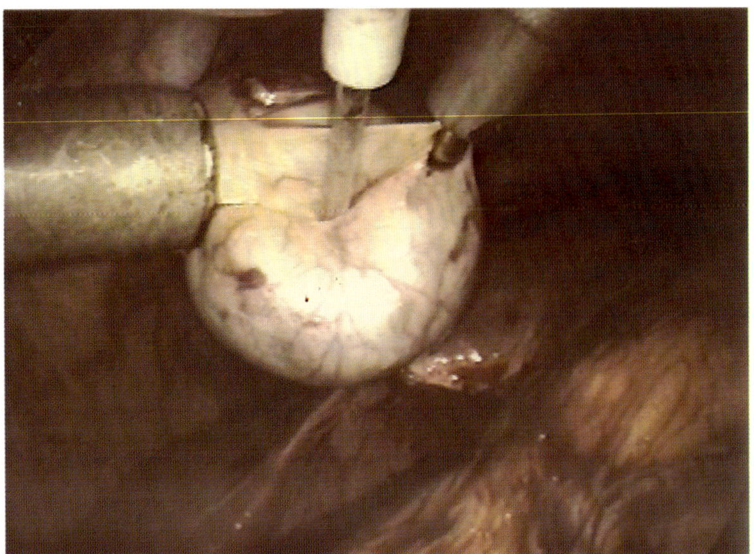

122

– A tense and filled gallbladder may
  have to be punctured and aspirated
  percutaneously

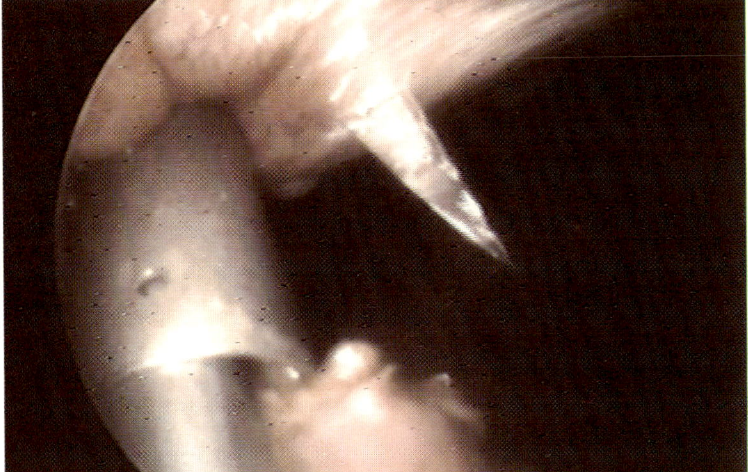

123

– For the gentle extraction of larger
  stones, the umbilical incision is dilated

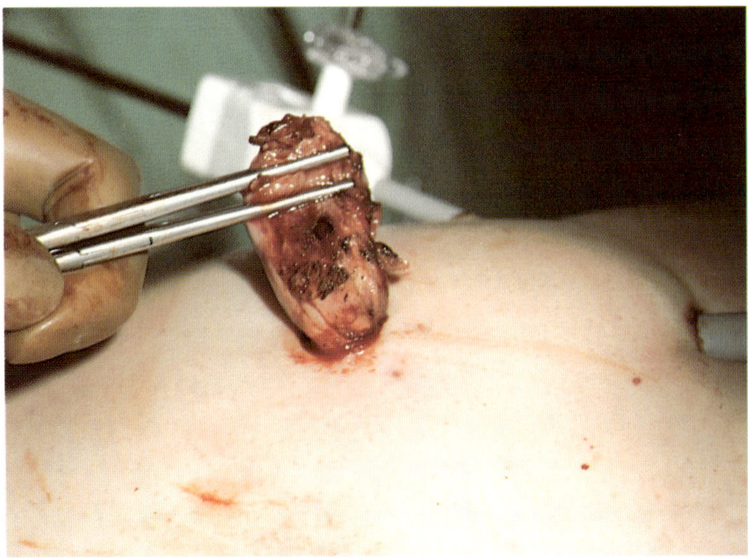

124

– After extraction through the umbilical incision, this port is temporarily
  closed with two towel clamps to
  maintain the pneumoperitoneum

## Irrigation and Hemostasis
(Figs. **125–127**)

– The liver is elevated with the palpation rod or with a grasping forceps
inserted via the lateral trocar

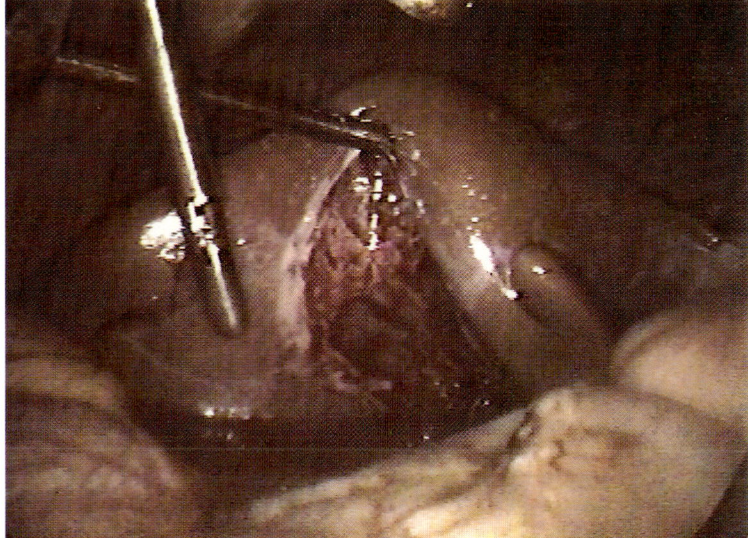

– Irrigation of the gallbladder bed is
followed by hemostasis with electrocautery and possibly the introduction of a hemostatic agent

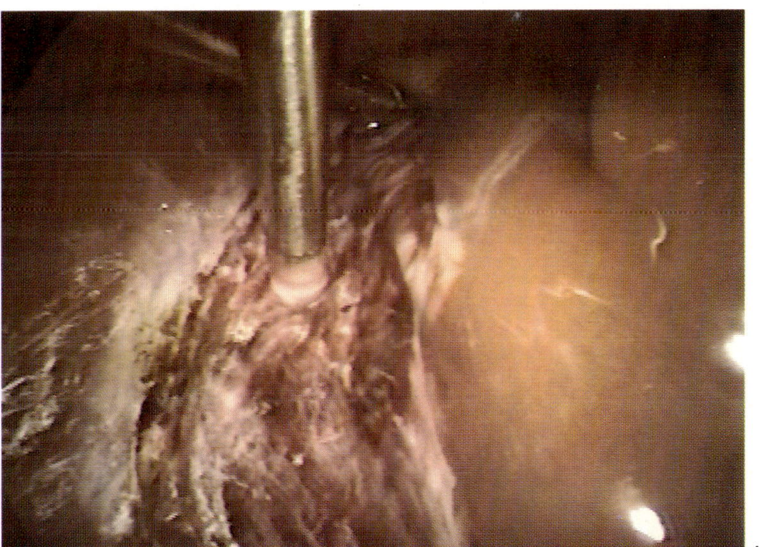

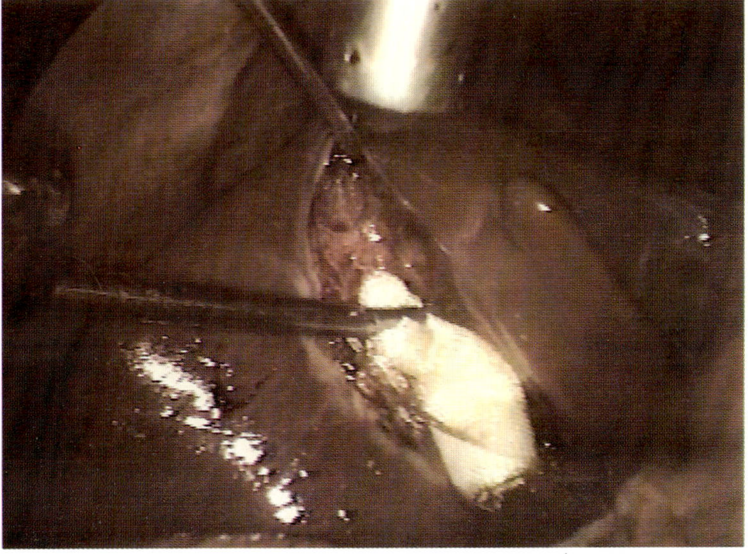

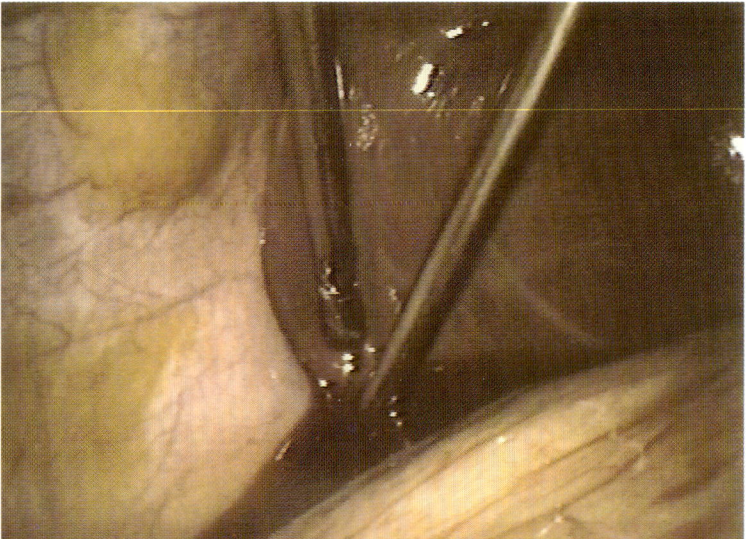

128

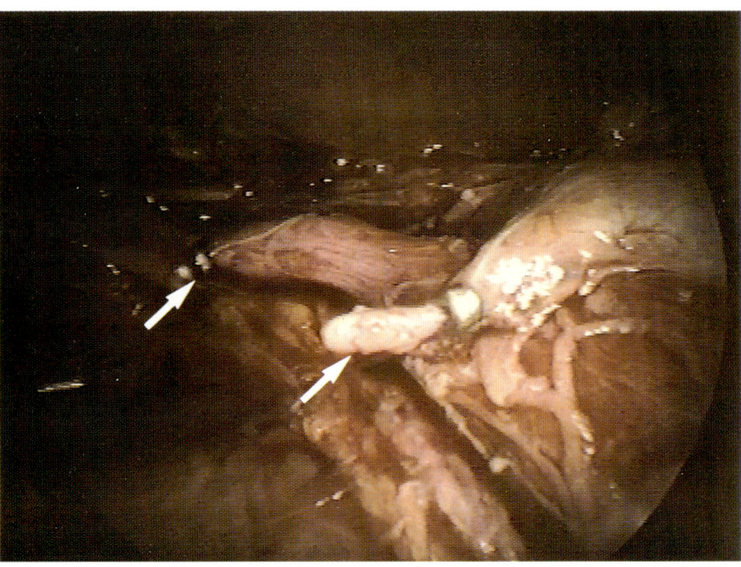

129

(Figs. **128, 129**)

– Blood clots and irrigation fluid below the diaphragm and below the liver are aspirated

– Final inspection of the stumps of the cystic duct and artery concludes this phase of the operation

## Drainage and Wound Closure
(Figs. **130–132**)

- If there is danger of blood or bile oozing, a soft silicone tube (5 mm) is inserted through the lateral trocar
- The tip of the tube is grasped with a forceps

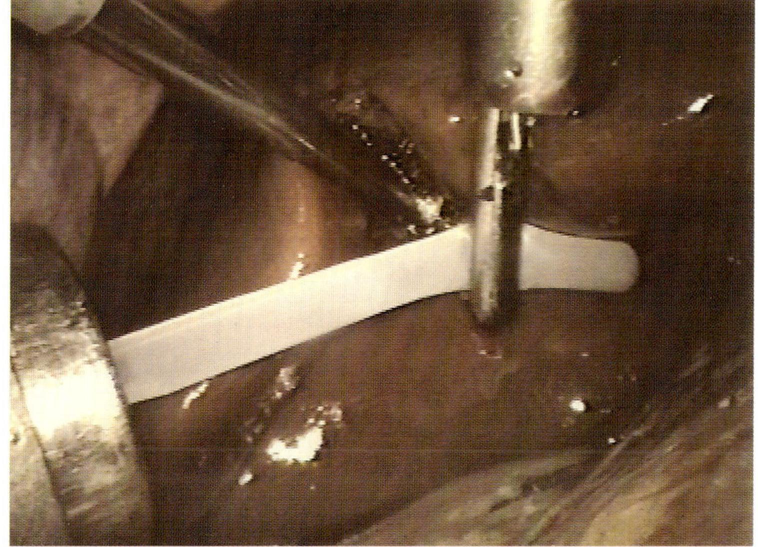

**130**

- The tip of the drain is placed anterior to the epiploic foramen

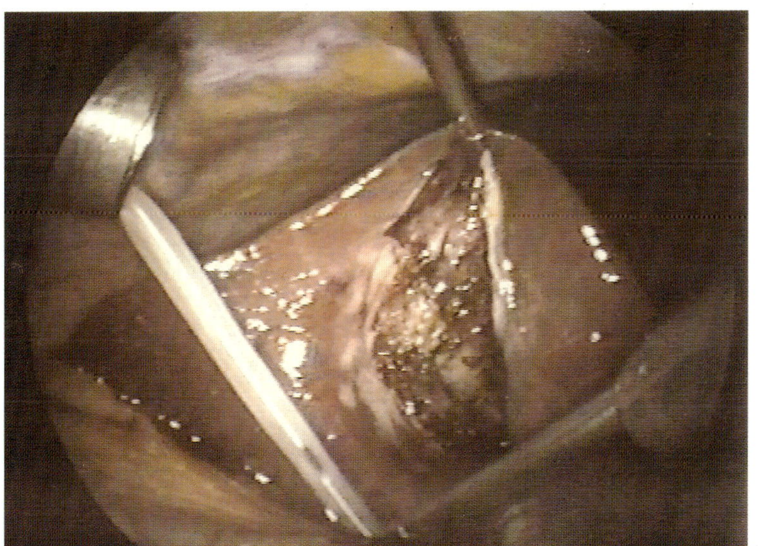

**131**

- The trocars are withdrawn under endoscopic vision *(watch out for omental tip herniation and bleeding from the puncture channel!)*
- Release of pneumoperitoneum
- Suture closure of the gap in the fascia in the area of the dilated incision or of the 20-mm trocar port
- Suture of skin

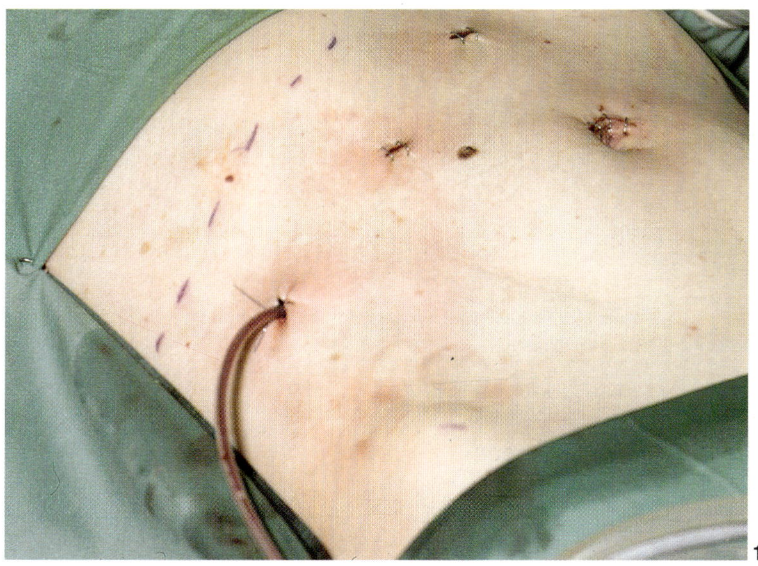

**132**

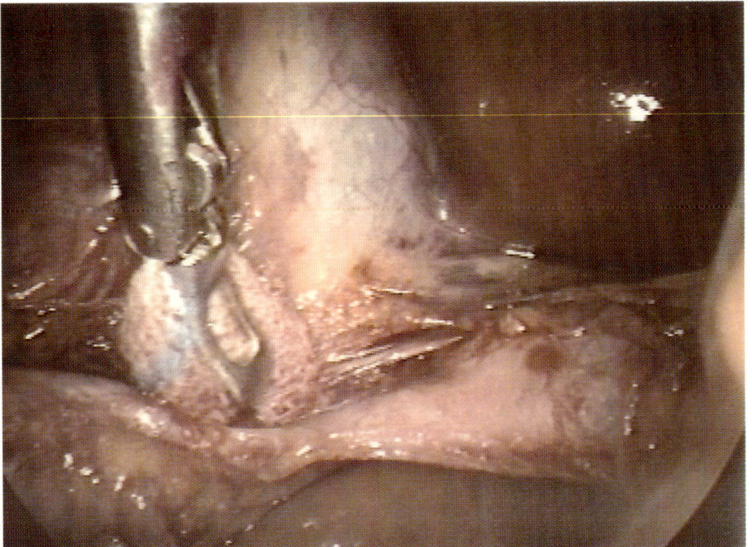

133

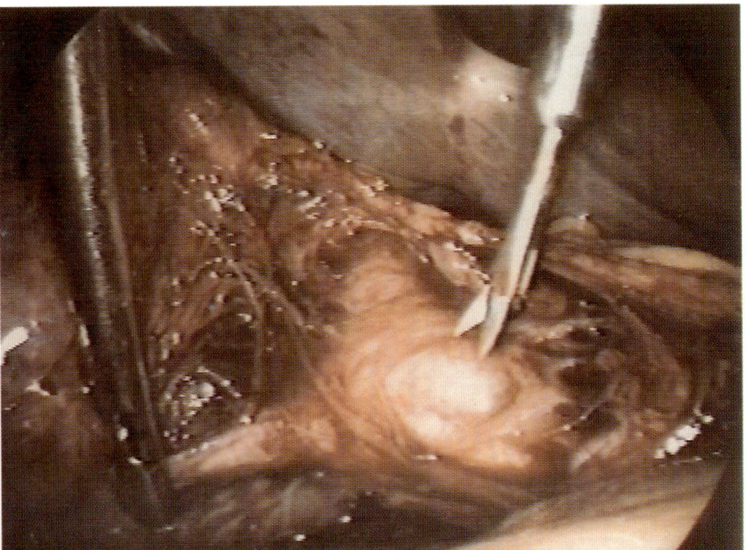

134

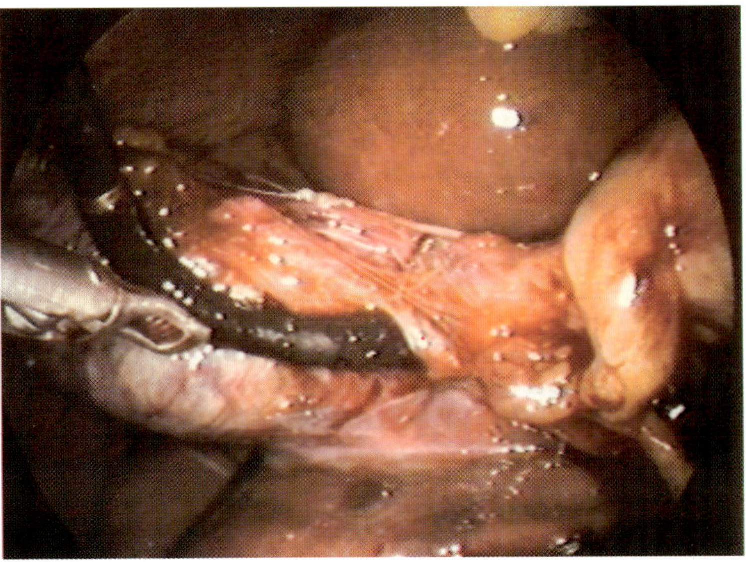

135

## Choledochotomy and Insertion of T-Tube

### Choledochotomy, Choledochoscopy
(Figs. **133–135**)

- See also the chapter on Indications
- Intraoperative cholangiography reveals a choledochal calculus
- An additional paramedian incision is made 10 mm to the left, under the costal arch, and an additional operating trocar, 11 mm, is introduced under endoscopic vision
- The common bile duct is dissected free

- A longitudinal incision (3 mm) is made in the common bile duct with microscissors, at the level of the junction with the cystic duct

- A 3-mm cholangioscope is inserted through the trocar in the midclavicular port and directed into the common bile duct

(Figs. **136–138**)

– Inspection of the hepatic duct
– Inspection of the common bile duct
  and the papilla
– Entry into the duodenum

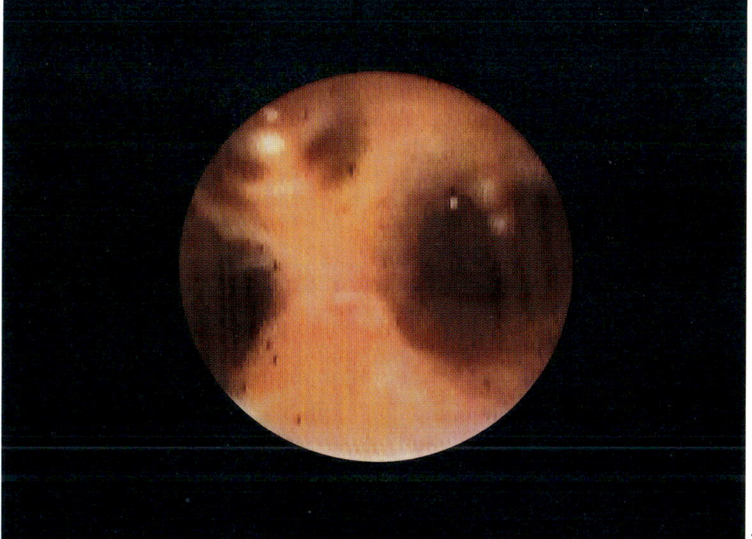

– Calculi are flushed out via the choledochotomy

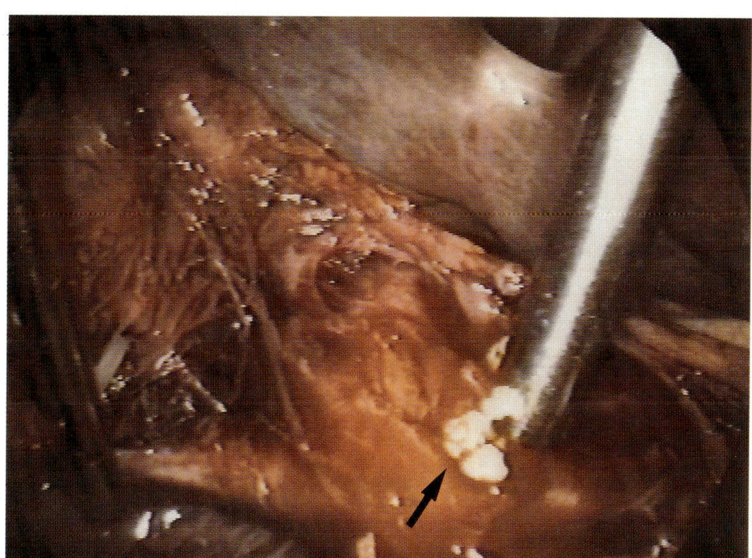

– A 3-mm T-tube is inserted through
  the left paramedian 11-mm operating trocar

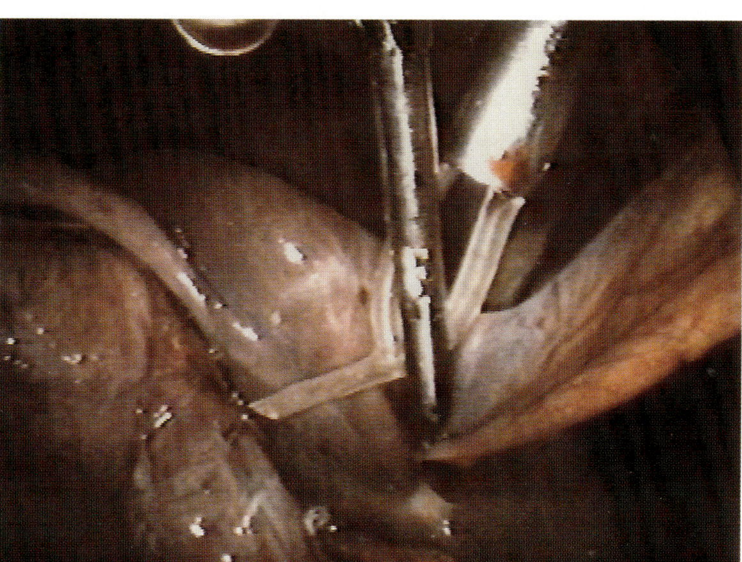

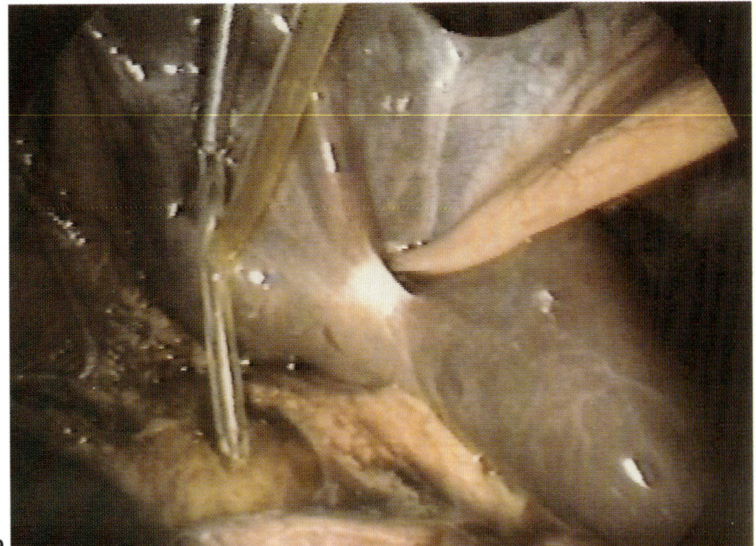

**139**

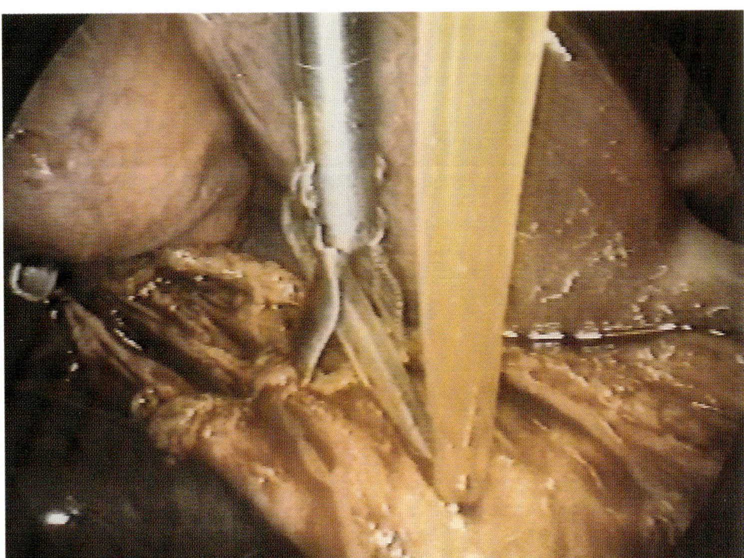

**140**

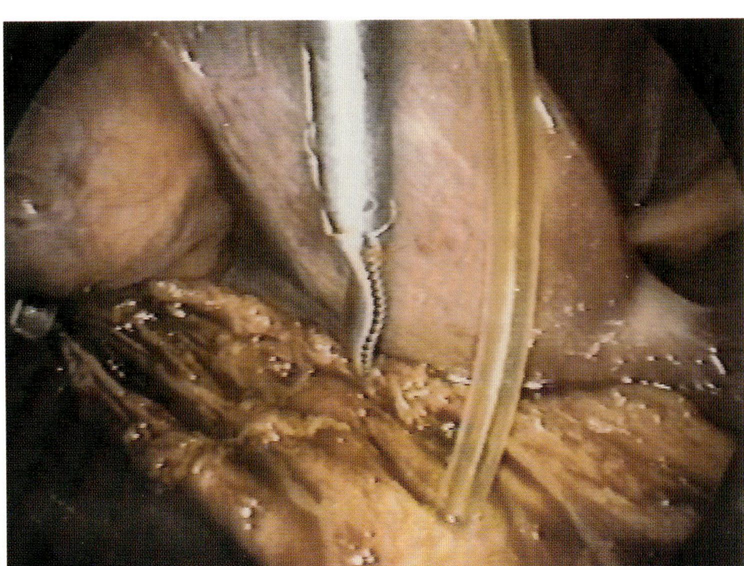

**141**

## Insertion of T-Drain
(Figs. **139—141**)

– The limbs are grasped with atraumatic grasping forceps and placed in the bile duct

## Closure of Choledochotomy
(Figs. **142–147**)

– Insertion of suture through right paramedian 11-mm trocar

– The needle is grasped with a needle holder, and the choledochotomy is closed with a continuous suture

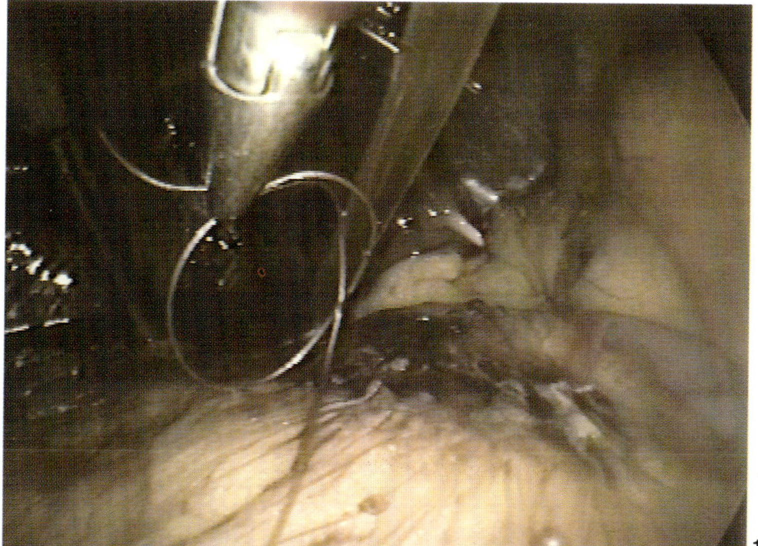

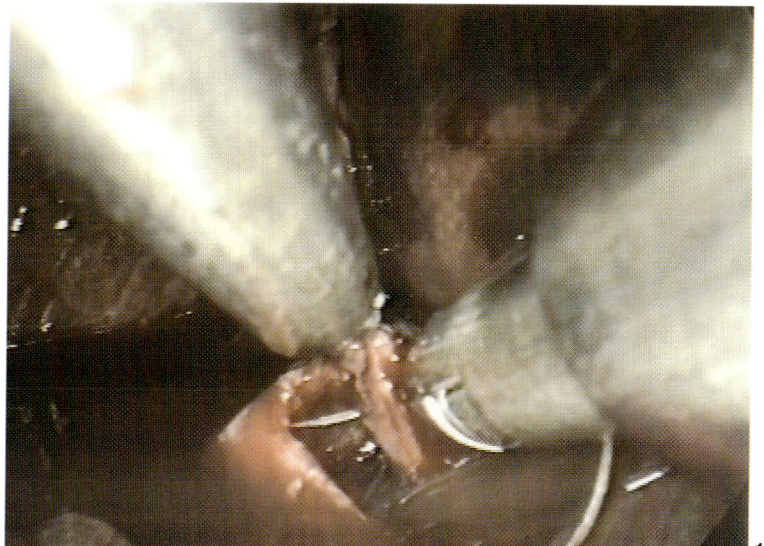

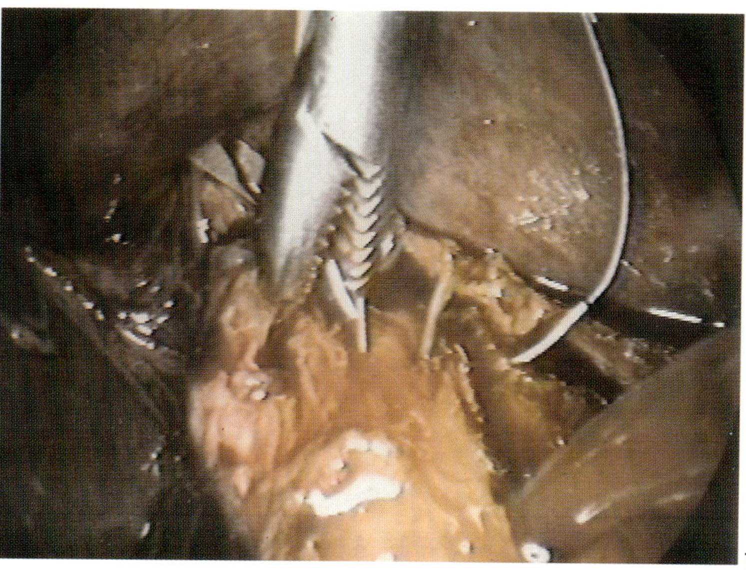

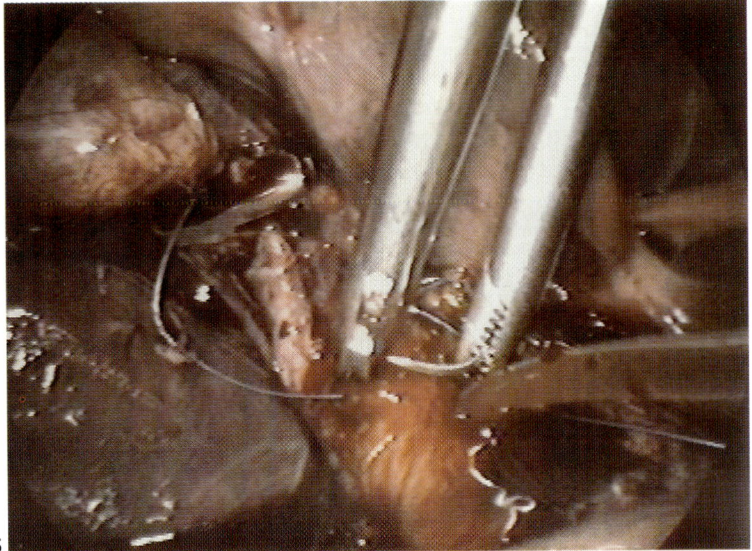

145

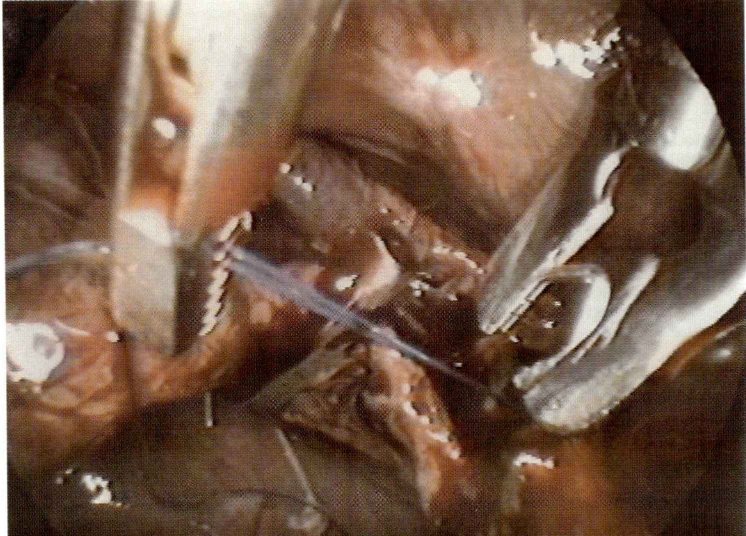

146

- Insertion of the clip applicator through the right paramedian 11-mm trocar and immobilization of suture ends with titanium clips
- A catheter is passed for the introduction of fibrin via the midclavicular 5.5-mm trocar
- Fibrin glue is applied to the choledochotomy
- A control cholangiography is performed via the T-tube (residual stone? leak?)
- Cholecystectomy

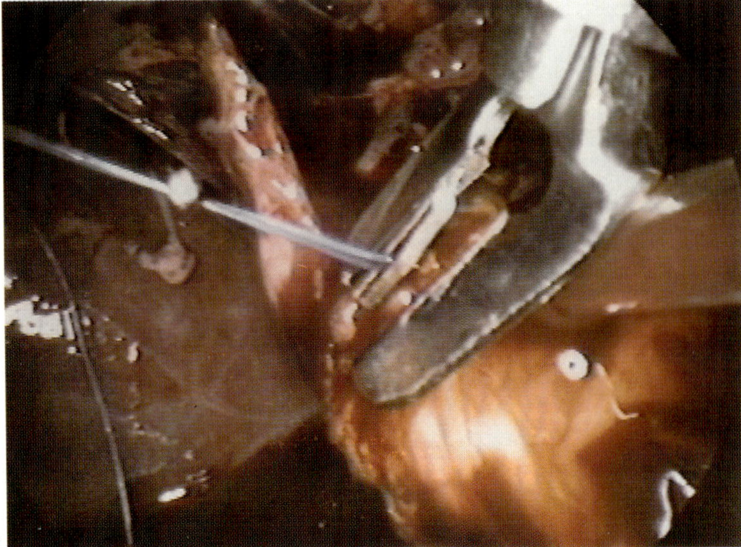

147

# Adhesiolysis

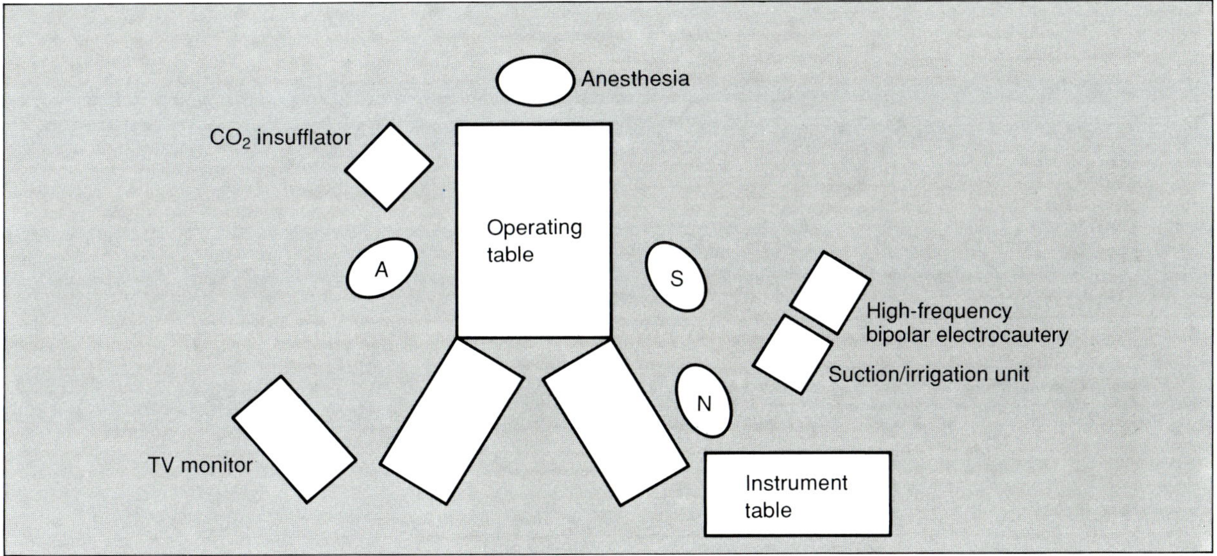


**148**

## Disposition of Equipment and Position of Surgical Team
(Fig. **148**)

- The surgeon (S) stands on the patient's left or right side, depending on the location of the anticipated adhesions
- The assistant (A) stands facing the surgeon
- The surgical nurse (N) and the instrument table are at the foot and to the left of the patient
- The TV monitor and the CO$_2$ insufflator are placed in the surgeon's line of vision
- The camera is operated by the surgeon

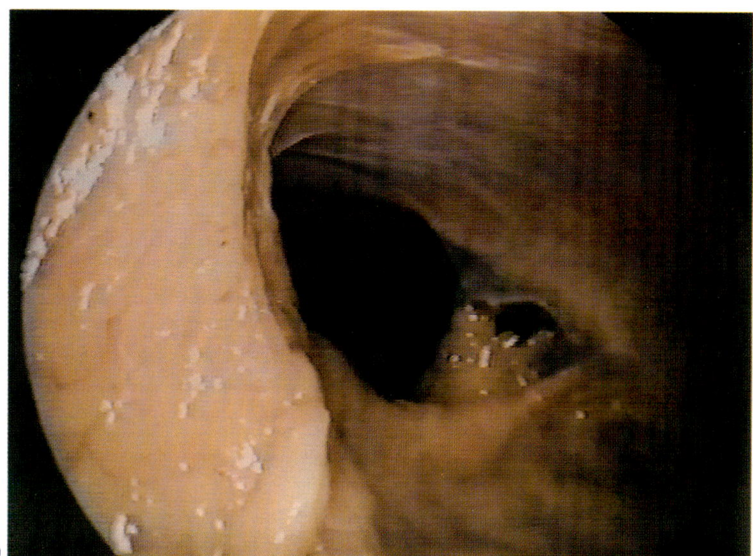

**149**

## Laparoscopic Trocar and Exploration
(Figs **149–151**)

- The laparoscopic trocar is inserted under endoscopic vision using the Semm technique
- Alternatively, a minilaparotomy is performed and the peritoneum sealed with a pursestring suture
- Visual exploration of the abdominal cavity

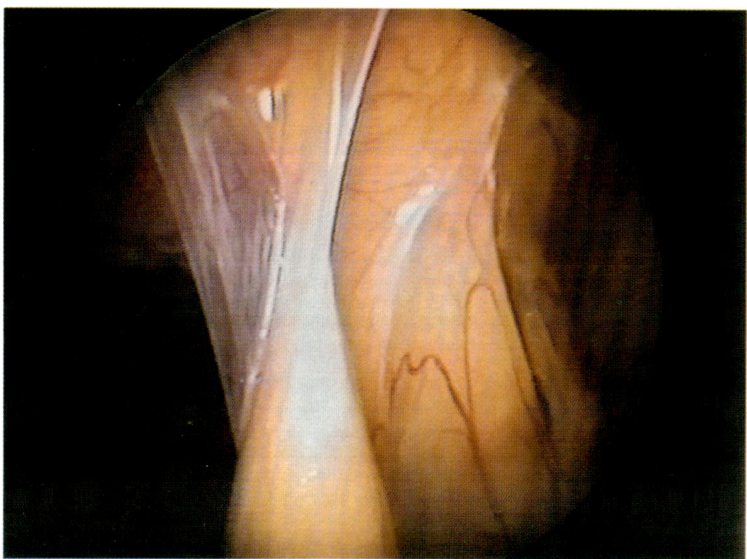

**150**

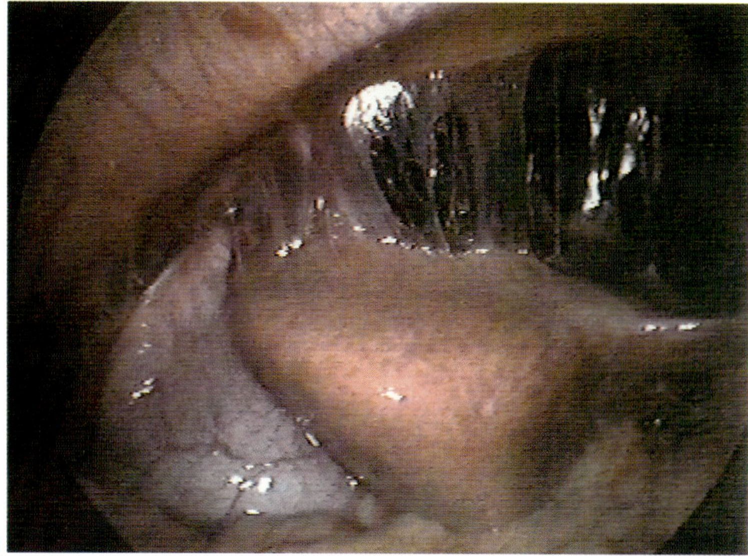

**151**

(Figs. **152–154**)

- Two additional operating trocars are introduced: a 5.5-mm trocar (grasping forceps, coagulating forceps, and Roeder endoloop) and an 11-mm trocar (grasping forceps, dissecting swab, clip applicator)
- The localization of the incisions for the operating trocars depends on the preceding operations. As a general rule, the quadrant of the abdomen opposite to a previous operation site will be chosen
- The surgeon has a choice between the lysis of adhesions by drying electrocautery followed by transection or by sharp dissection and hemostasis as indicated, if the local status favors this approach

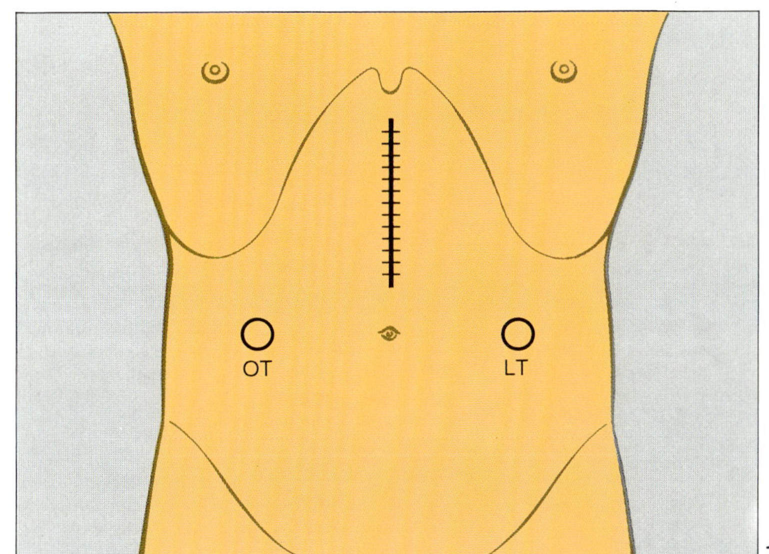



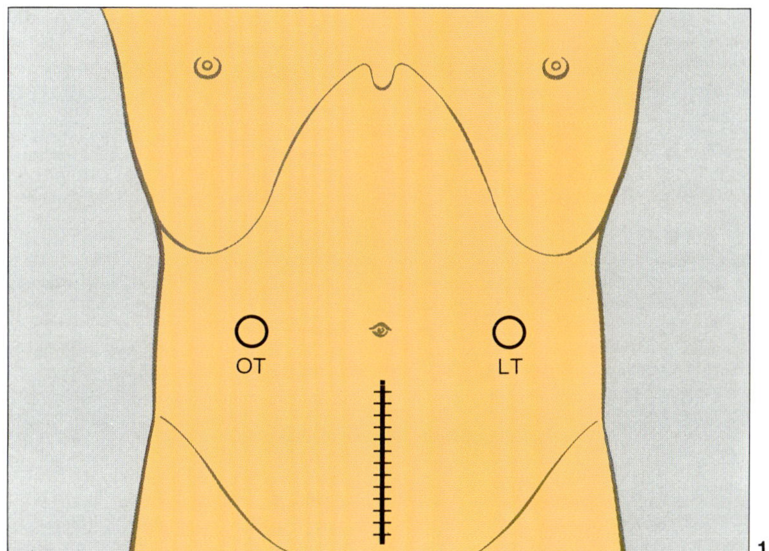



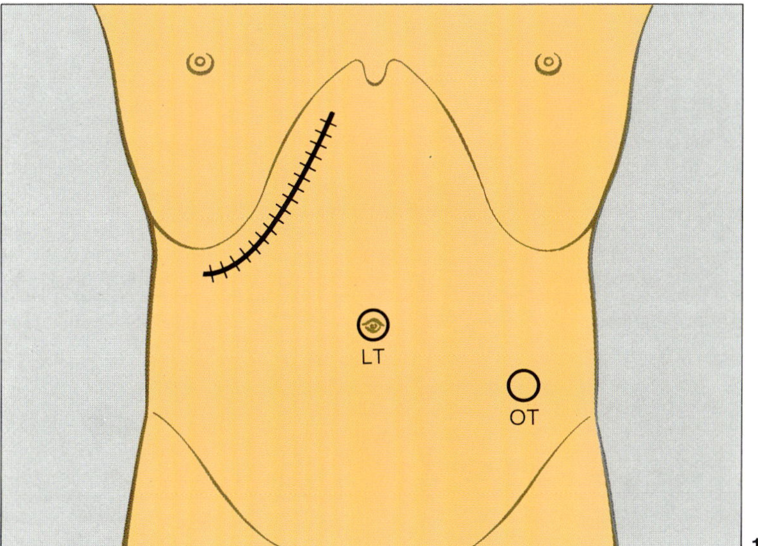

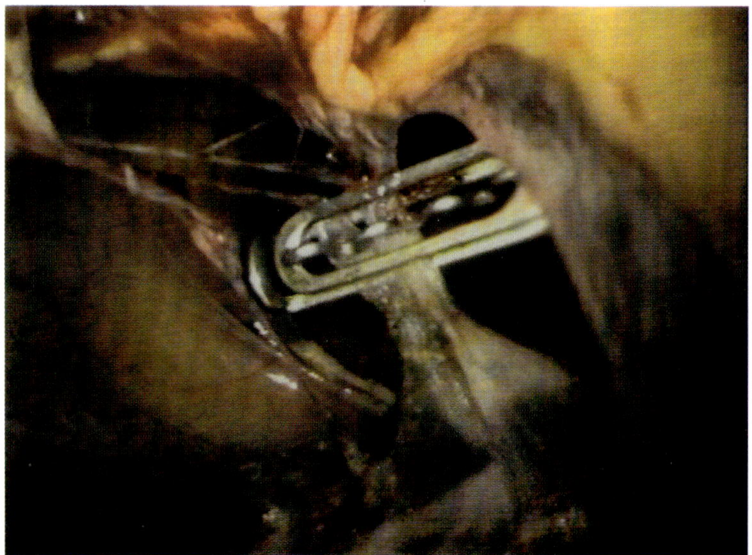

**155**

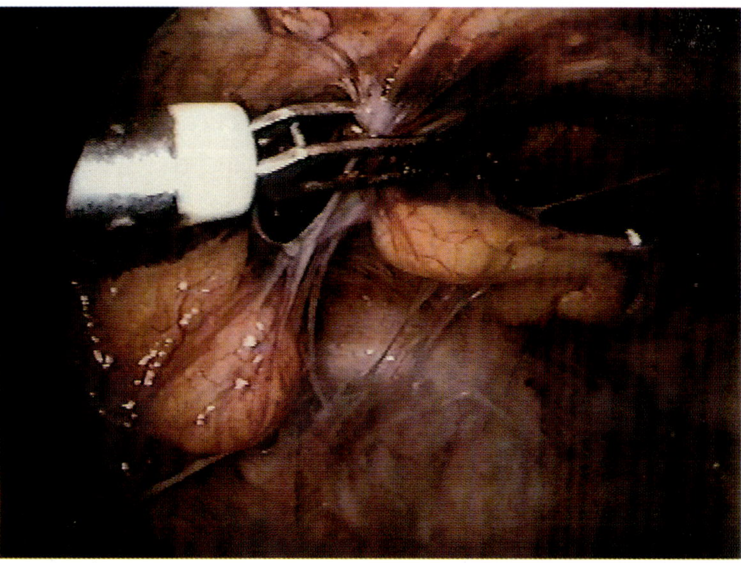

**156**

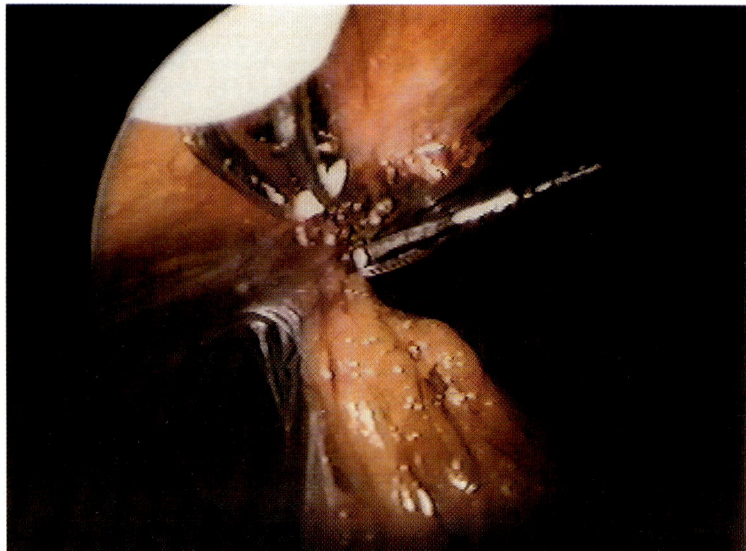

**157**

## Dry Adhesiolysis
(Figs. **155—157**)

- The adhesions are put under tension with the atraumatic grasping forceps

- The tightened bands are desiccated with the high-frequency bipolar coagulating forceps and then sharply divided

- Adhesions between the parietal peritoneum and the visceral peritoneum require stretching of the intestine with dissecting forceps and sharp transection close to the abdominal wall

## Adhesiolysis by Sharp Dissection
(Figs. **158–160**)

- The adhesions are drawn tight by traction with an atraumatic grasping forceps

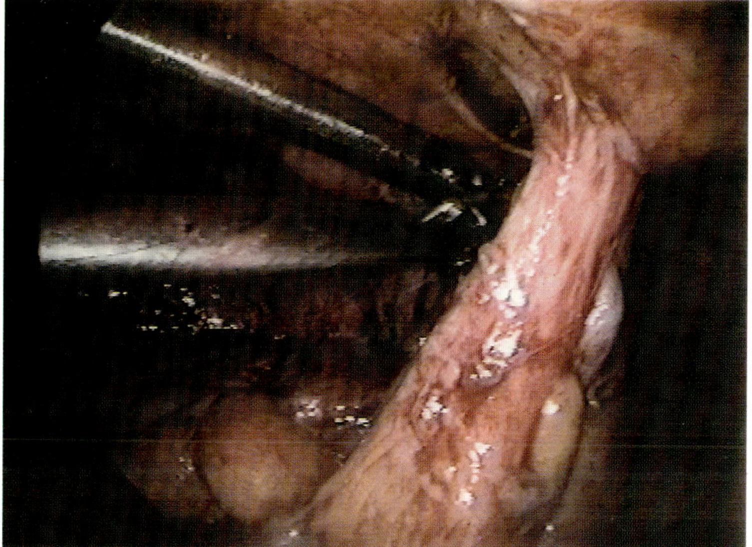

**158**

- They are divided with scissors close to the abdominal wall

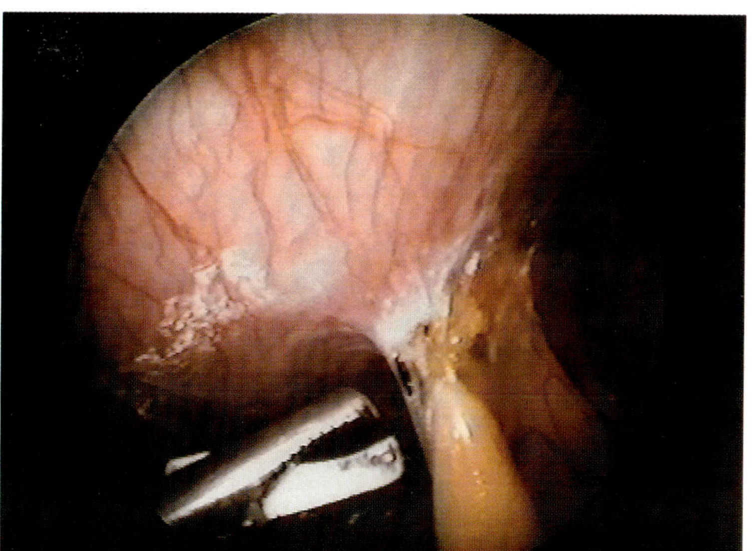

**159**

- A Roeder endoloop is opened with atraumatic grasping forceps and the bleeding ablation site is grasped through the ring of the loop
- Ligation and division of the suture
- Bleeding parietal adhesion sites may have to be coagulated with a bipolar grasping forceps *(watch out for the intestine)*

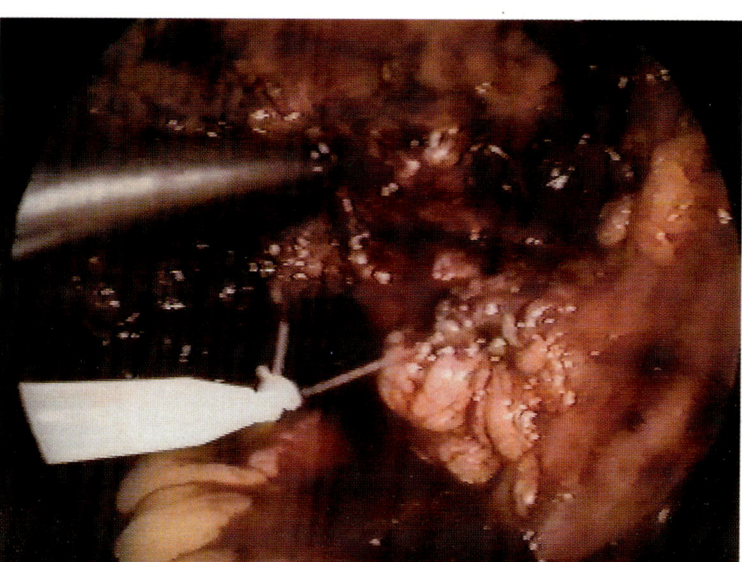

**160**

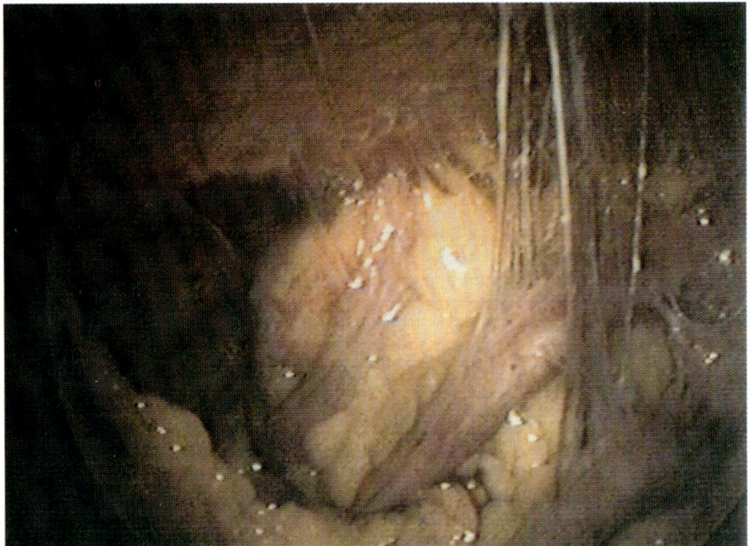

161

## Adhesions between Intestinal Loops

- Adhesions between intestinal loops are put under tension with an atraumatic grasping forceps, coagulated, and sharply divided *(watch out for heat damage to the intestinal wall!)*
- Accidental lesions of the intestinal wall that open the lumen should be closed conventionally via minilaparotomy

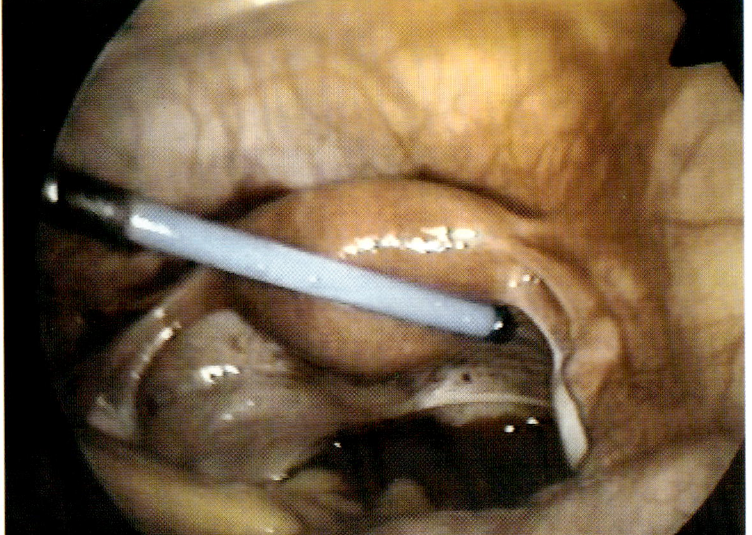

162

## Conclusion of Adhesiolysis

- Final inspection of dissection area
- Irrigation and aspiration of secretions
- Placement of a silicone drain in the space of Douglas for oozing
- Withdrawal of trocar sheaths under vision

# Postoperative Care

The size of the wound(s) in the abdominal wall and the nature of the intra-abdominal procedure are critical in determining the postoperative course and the patient's subjective well-being. Both factors need to be considered in the aftercare that follows any abdominal operation. The small incisions required in interventional laparoscopy and the reduced intra-abdominal trauma made possible by the absence of eventration and intestinal manipulation are associated with a more rapid return to normal by the patient.

However, the early return of well-being and the lack of patient awareness of "incisional" disease should not make us forget that the intra-abdominal healing process is essentially organ-related. Independently of the type of operation performed, postoperative care begins while the patient is still on the operating table, when the stomach tube and possibly a bladder catheter are withdrawn. After diagnostic laparoscopy, aftercare is limited to measures required solely by the anesthesia. The patient is observed in the ward for several hours (blood pressure and pulse). Any wound or shoulder pain that may be experienced due to incompletely absorbed $CO_2$ lodged below the diaphragm (Riedel 1981) generally remains within the range of tolerable discomfort or can easily be controlled by the administration of analgesics. After recovery from the anesthetic drug action, the patient may be discharged, possibly even on the same day. The necessary wound care can be carried out on an ambulatory basis and is completed with removal of the skin sutures or steristrips on the 7th or 8th postoperative day (Fig. **163**). Patients who have undergone operative laparoscopies, such as extensive adhesiolysis, appendectomy, or cholecystectomy, receive parenteral alimentation on the day of the operation. Mobilization begins during the evening of the same day. Oral feeding is started on the first postoperative day with tea and toast. If the course is unremarkable, the patient may have light meals on the next day. The choice of procedure regarding indwelling catheters is no different from that for laparotomy. Postoperative wound pain following laparoscopic operations can be controlled by the oral administration of analgesics. Shoulder pain may occasionally persist for as long as 1 week after the operation. In an uncomplicated course, the postoperative hospital stay is at present 1−3 days after laparoscopic appendectomy and 1−4 days after laparoscopic cholecystectomy.

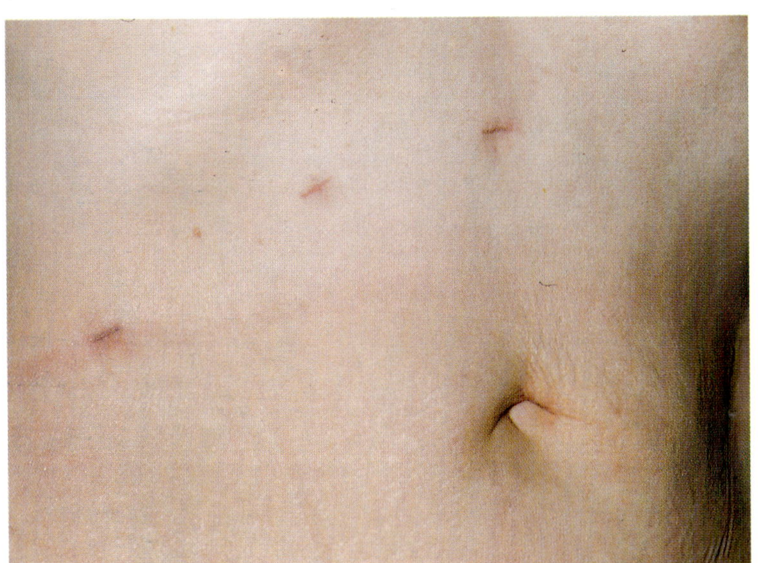

Fig. **163**    Wound healing on the eighth day after laparoscopic cholecystectomy

# Complications and Their Treatment

In the hands of experienced surgeons, laparoscopy has been a safe and reliable method. A mortality rate of $0-0.3\%$ has been reported from large series in internal medicine (Brühl 1966), gynecology (Semm 1979), and surgery (Zimmerman 1982).

Morbidity and mortality vary according to age, associated disease, and the surgeon's experience. Complications that arise are generally easy to control; a few, however, are acutely life-threatening. Iatrogenic complications are caused mostly by the use of inadequate techniques and lack of experience. This underscores the need for the systematic training of surgeons practicing laparoscopy. The principal intraoperative and postoperative complications and their management are described below.

## Intraoperative Complications

### Faulty Induction of Pneumoperitoneum

Gas insufflation with an extraperitoneally lying needle due to tangential or excessively deep puncture may be associated with emphysema of the skin, the preperitoneal space, omentum, and mediastinum. This complicates the examination but has no serious consequences. The gas is absorbed by the body without sequelae.

### Puncture of a Hollow Viscus

As a rule, puncture of a hollow abdominal organ with the Verres needle, detectable by the escape of gas via natural channels and orifices or by an asymmetrical induction of the pneumoperitoneum with unilateral elevation of the abdominal wall, generally has no dramatic effects. After the selection of a new puncture site and proper induction of the pneumoperitoneum, the earlier puncture site should be carefully inspected to evaluate the extent of the injury. Small penetrations with no escape of intestinal contents will heal in response to nonoperative measures such as gastric intubation, fasting, and antibiotic protection. Larger injuries from which intestinal contents escape have to be treated by laparotomy and sutured closing.

### Inadvertent Puncture of Vessels

Gas embolism is a potential risk. This complication has rarely been reported since $CO_2$ began to be used for induction of the pneumoperitoneum (Root et al. 1978). However, if gas embolism is suspected, the patient should immediately by placed in the head down and left lateral position. The diagnosis should be confirmed by cardiopulmonary monitoring with a Swan–Ganz catheter and Doppler sonography.

If the puncture of a vessel becames apparent by the aspiration of blood and is not associated with a rapidly developing picture of clinical shock due to hypovolemia, in which case immediate laparotomy is mandatory, the laparoscopy may be "routinely" continued at first. However, repeated inspection of the puncture site and the usually developing hematoma is imperative. If an increase in the size of the hematoma or clinical shock should supervene during the course of laparoscopy, laparotomy is indicated.

## Laceration of the Vena Cava

It is important to understand that the pressure of the pneumoperitoneum exerts some degree of compression on hollow organs, especially the low flow, low pressure inferior vena cava and its contributaries. This tamponade between the posterior peritoneum and the firm muscles and bones of the trunk could easily hide a critical laceration of the inferior vena cava or iliac veins, even while the laparoscopic operation is "routinely" in progress.

If such an event is suspected, blood and fluids for volume replacement should be readied, control venous lines and monitoring with a Swan–Ganz catheter should be established before the pneumoperitoneum is evacuated and the pressure released, while already positioned trocars are left in place. Careful observation of clinical and physiological (Swan–Ganz) signs of hypovolemia, enlargement of abdominal girth, blood spontaneously evacuated through the trocars, and early laparoscopic observation of bleeding or an enlarging peritoneal hematoma after the pneumoperitoneum has been reestablished should lead to a wide laparotomy and control of the venous injury.

## Trocar Injury

Bleeding into the abdominal wall due to injury of a vessel by insertion of the laparoscopic or operating trocar can be controlled by compression. By contrast, injury of a hollow organ by the trocar is a serious complication which requires immediate laparotomy. It is advisable to leave the trocar in place if the intestine (Fig. **164**) or the stomach have been entered accidentally. Through a small midline laparotomy, the perforation site can then be rapidly located and oversewn. Injury of the parenchymatous organs as well as of larger vessels with the trocar necessitate immediate· laparotomy, as described above.

## Hemorrhage

Hemorrhage occurring in the course of the dissection (Fig. **165**) can be rapidly located thanks to the good visibility and the magnification afforded by the lens systems. Bleeding is treated either by coagulation or by application of the Roeder endoloop or of hemochips. Uncontrollable hemorrhage, however, calls for prompt laparotomy.

## Lost Foreign Bodies

Lost swabs (Fig. **166**), individual gallstones, tissue parts, or clips should be retrieved and removed laparoscopically. Lost clips that cannot be found may have to be left behind.

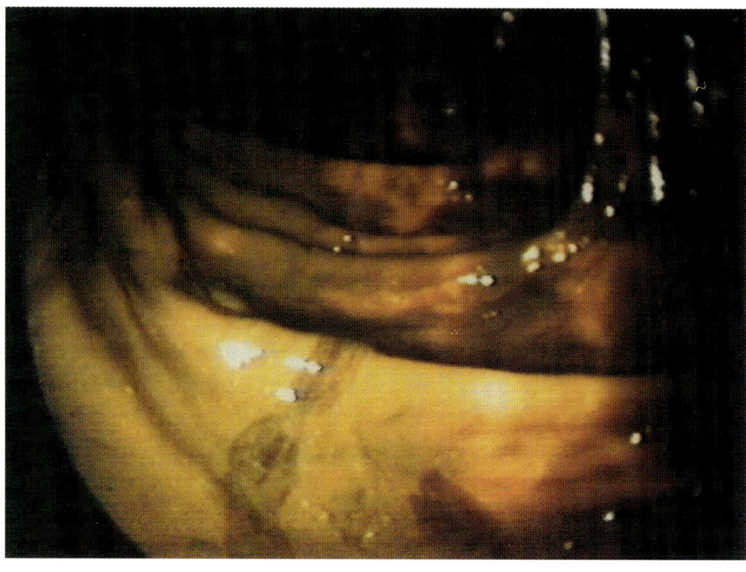

Fig. **164**   Complication due to insertion of the laparoscopic trocar: The colonic lumen is visible after placement of the laparoscope and camera

Fig. **165**  Complication during dissection: blood spurting from the appendiceal artery

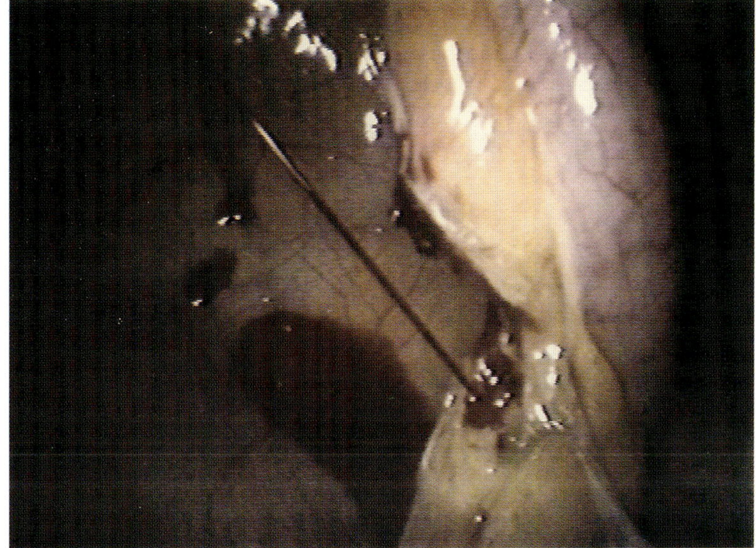

Fig. **166**  Complication during iodine disinfection of appendiceal stump: loss of swab

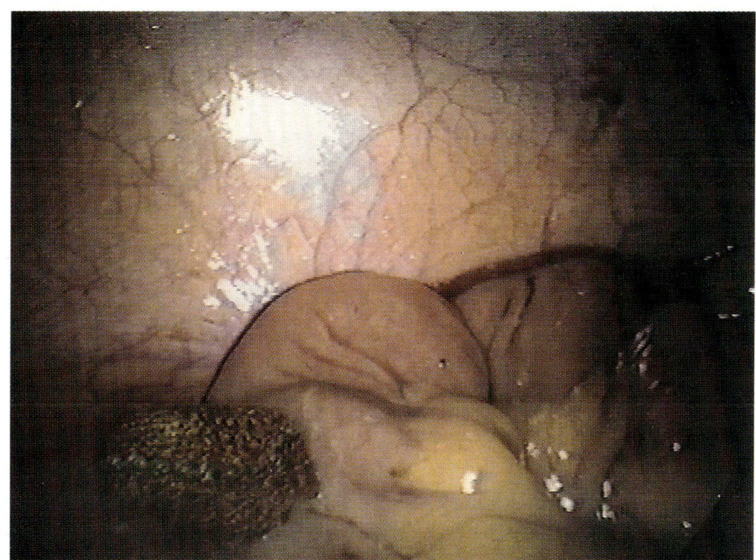

Fig. **167**  Complication during closure of the appendiceal stump: escape of feces into the abdominal cavity after slippage of the Roeder loop

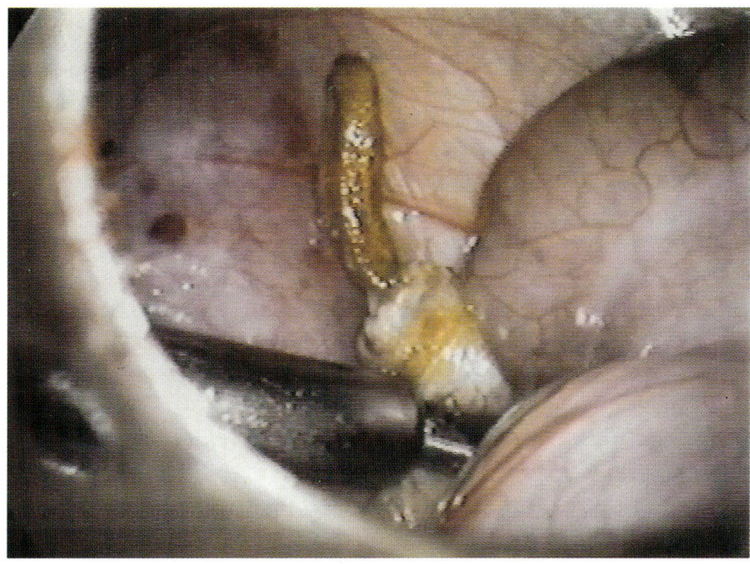

## Intestinal Injury

The use of high-frequency coagulation, as in appendectomy, for example, entails the risk of damage to the cecal cul-de-sac and adjacent intestinal loops. Keeping a safe distance and good exposure are indispensable. Incomplete stump closure or a slipped endoloop causing escape of feces into the abdominal cavity (Fig. **167**) as well as any accidental intestinal lesion require immediate attention via laparotomy.

## Bile Duct Injury

The most important complications of laparoscopic cholecystectomy are injuries of the gallbladder and bile ducts, oozing of blood from the liver bed, and arterial hemorrhage. Small lesions of the gallbladder due to the dissection can be treated by tangential clip application or use of the endoloop (Fig. **168**). An attempt should always be made to close the perforation site. Potential infection risks are posed by the escape of bile and by stones that have been missed. Free bile should therefore be completely aspirated from the peritoneal cavity, and individual stones can be extracted with the aid of grasping forceps. If there is the slightest suspicion of injury to the bile ducts, the operation has be to continued with the abdomen opened and the bile duct explored if necessary. The danger of an iatrogenic bile duct lesion, particularly under anatomically uncertain conditions, underscores the need for intraoperative radiological exploration of the bile ducts and image documentation.

## Rebleeding

The most common bleeding source is the cystic artery. Rebleeding from the appendicular artery occurs less frequently. Causes of rebleeding comprise imperfect identification during dissection, anatomical variations, and slippage of the hemostatic clips. If there is bleeding from the cystic artery, the site should be clearly exposed after aspiration of the blood clots and the stump grasped and closed with a clip. The multitude of anatomical variations entailing the risk of erroneous closure of the right hepatic artery requires its unequivocal identification as well. In case of doubt, an open exploration is preferable. Oozing of blood from the liver bed can be

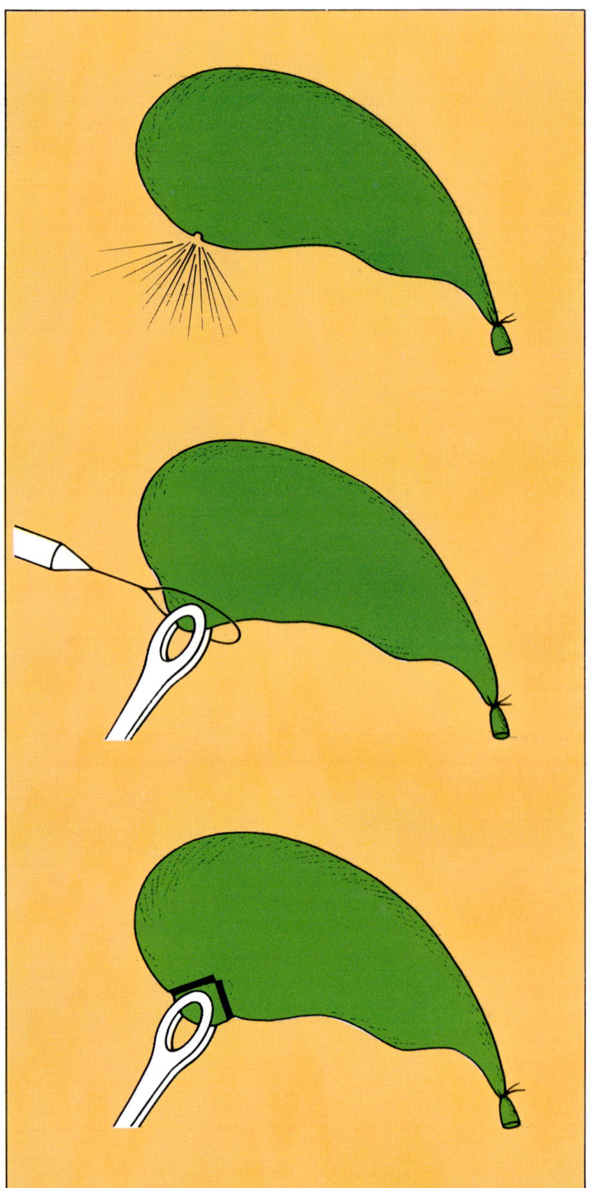

Fig. **168**  Complication during dissection of the gallbladder: perforation and escape of bile. This may be closed either by tangential clip application or with the Roeder loop

controlled by electrocoagulation. In some cases, a hemostatic agent may also be placed in the gallbladder bed.

## Postoperative Complications

Essentially, the only postoperative complication specific to the technique is shoulder pain due to incomplete evacuation of $CO_2$ from the abdominal cavity. Wound infections in the umbilical region are rare and avoidable by careful disinfection of the umbilical fossa. Omental or intestinal incarceration results from overly hasty withdrawal of the trocars while the pneumoperitoneum has not yet been completely eliminated. This complication can be prevented if the trocars are brought out under vision and the gas is completely released before the laparoscopic trocar is removed.

The incidence of operation-specific complications such as rebleeding, bile duct injury during cholecystectomy, and stump incompetence in appendectomy with regional abscess does not seem any higher than in conventional procedures. Their diagnosis and treatment do not differ fundamentally from those after conventional operative procedures. As a rule, laparotomy is unavoidable for the revision.

---

*Complications of Laparoscopic Operations*

*Induction of pneumoperitoneum:*
> Emphysema of skin, preperitoneal space, omentum and mediastinum
> Gas embolism
> Vessel puncture
> Puncture of a hollow organ (stomach, intestine, bladder)

*Insertion of trocars:*
> Perforation of a hollow organ (stomach, intestine, bladder)
> Injury of larger vessels (aorta, vena cava)
> Bleeding into abdominal wall
> Parenchymal injury

*Operation-specific:*
> Bleeding during dissection (appendicular artery, cystic artery, adhesions)
> Loss of foreign bodies (swabs, clips)
> Escape of intestinal contents (feces, bile, gallstone)
> Heat damage during coagulation (intestine, common bile duct, etc.)
> Gallbladder injury
> Slippage of ligatures or clips (e.g., appendiceal stump, cystic artery)

# Documentation of Records

## Operative Report

The introduction of the video technique into endoscopy has opened up new dimensions for medical documentation. The general possibility of visually recording the entire course of an operation does not relieve the surgeon of his fundamental obligation to provide a written operative report. Besides the customary comprehensive description of the operative course, it is important to record in writing a number of technical data, such as the level of the preselected intra-abdominal pressure, the type and quantity of the gas used for induction of the pneumoperitoneum, the diameter and localization of the trocars, and the type of current used for coagulation. In addition, it is helpful to cite separately in the operative report, besides the selected positioning mode, the safety tests that were carried out and their results. Retrieval of these routinely generated data is greatly facilitated by the supply of a special documentation form (Fig. **169**) for the laparoscopic operative report—comparable to the "pelviscopic operation report" proposed by Semm (1984)—including preprinted column headings and possibly a graph.

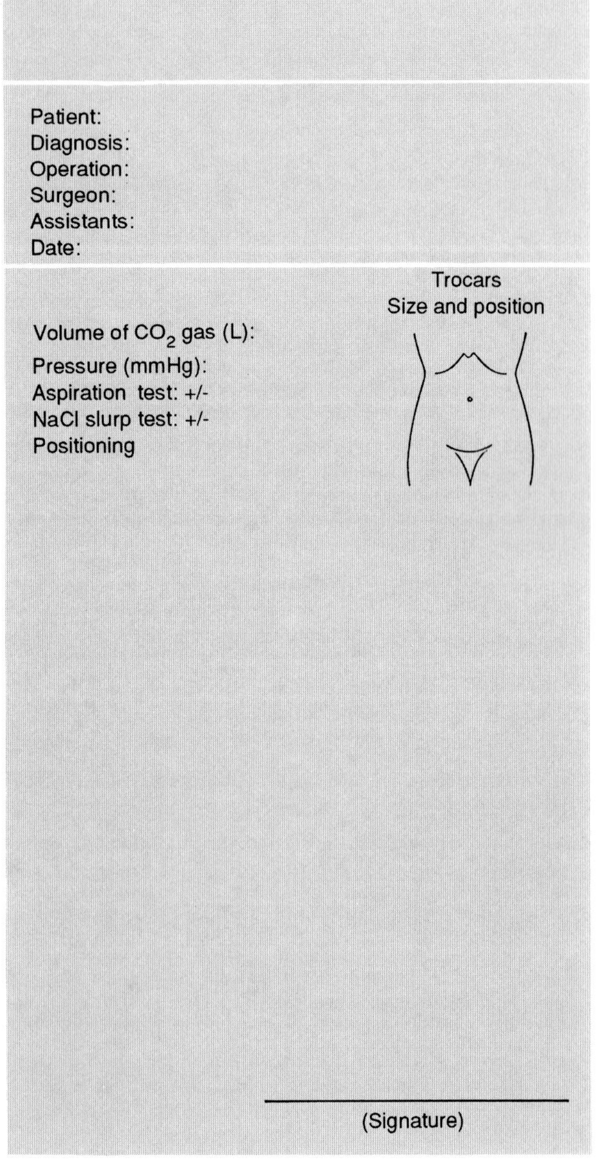


Fig. **169** Report form for written recording of laparoscopic procedures

## Monitor Transmission

Direct transmission of the image from the laparoscope to the TV monitor offers many advantages. First of all, the surgeon is relieved of the necessity of maintaining the tiring posture required to keep the eye fixed directly on the laparoscope. The laparoscopic site appears on the monitor in a large format (Fig. **170**) and thus becomes accessible for the first time not only to the surgeon but to the whole team. The lightweight miniaturized CCD-chip camera with high image resolution in combination with the powerful cold light sources permits precise anatomical orientation and exploration of the abdominal cavity as well as good documentation of the findings. Each step of the operation can be followed on the TV monitor under conditions comparable to daylight. The direct access of a large group of people to the image data leads to coordinated action by all those involved; the anesthetist, too, is kept informed of the status of the operation at all times. Image transmission to the monitor additionally provides an opportunity for direct training in laparoscopic procedures.

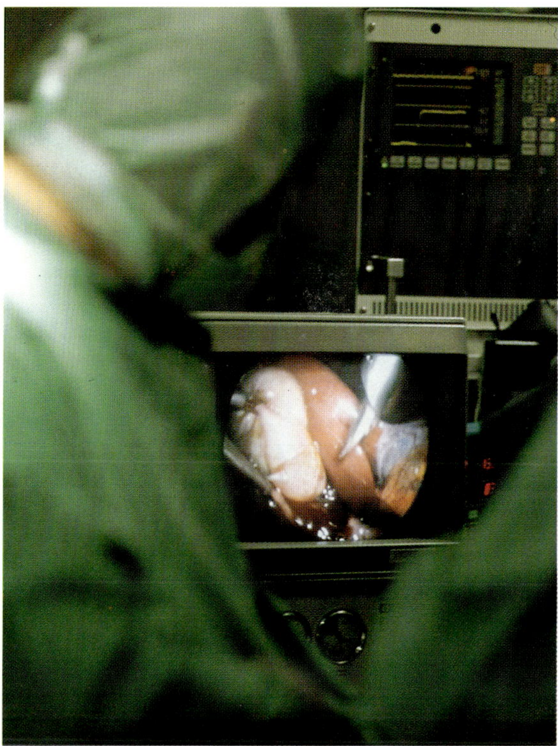

Fig. **170**   The monitor transmission shows an enlarged picture of the intra-abdominal site for the benefit of the whole surgical team

## Video Recording

Video recording for the purposes of documentation is already widely used in video endoscopy. It is an inexpensive, uncomplicated method of documentation. Complete operative sequences or selected sequences only may be stored as desired. This makes possible repeated demonstration of the pathological findings and retrospective analysis of the operation performed. Additionally, the pictorial material may be utilized for scientific presentations and training. For routine documentation, a VHS recorder is sufficient. The higher requirements of acuity and color quality for scientific documentation, on the other hand, can be met only by U-Matic or S-VHS tapes. The lower price of the S-VHS tapes has to be weighed against the currently more widespread use of the U-Matic system and the possibilities of reproduction that this implies.

## Disk Recorder and Video Printer

As an alternative to the video cassette, storage of important image sequences by means of a disk recorder is possible. With the use of two-sided floppy disks, as many as 37 000 individual images can be stored on one disk. This means a considerable saving of storage space and permits rapid retrieval of the data.

Selected sections can be called in at any time and printed out with the aid of a video printer, for example (Fig. **171**). These may be attached to the patient's records for documentation or passed on to the patient or his or her physician. The required image quality of the video printer should, in view of the as yet considerable differences in price, be made to conform to the actual purpose to be served (routine or scientific documentation).

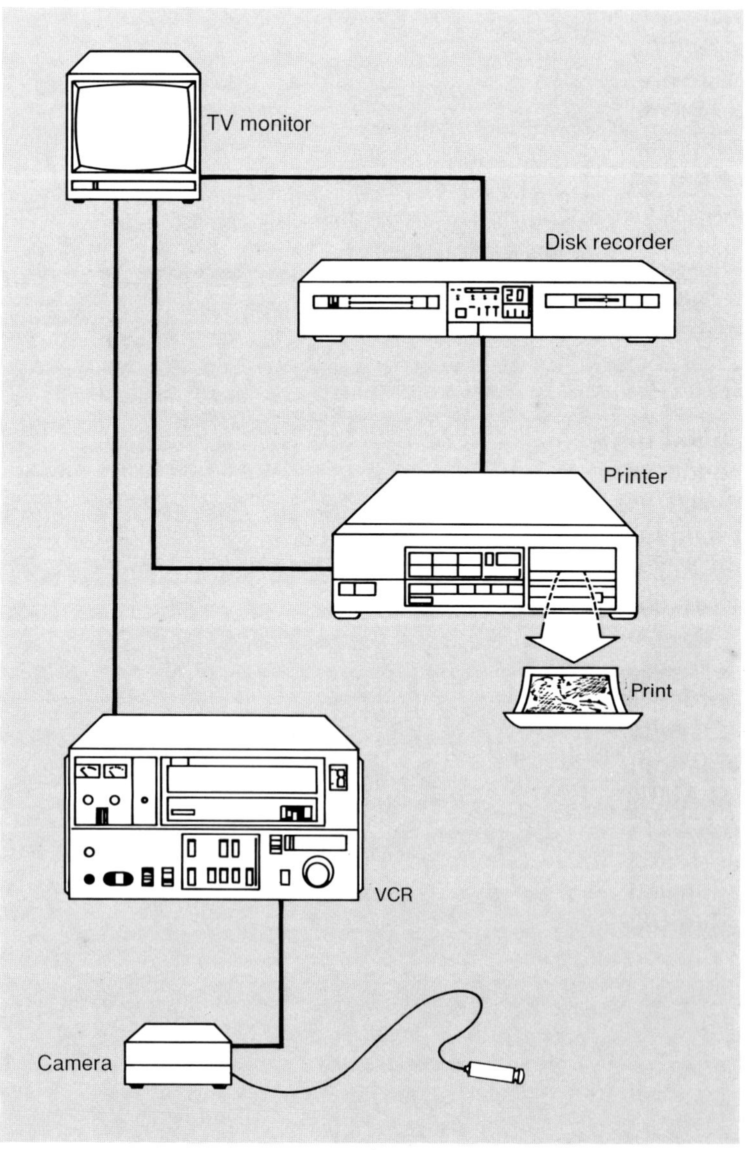


Fig. **171**   Schematic representation of a practical arrangement of various components for the documentation of the laparoscopic procedures

# Further Development of the Laparoscopic Instrumentation

An inadequate instrumentation often remains the limiting factor in the performance of new laparoscopic procedures. New developments in the field of insufflators with automatic pressure equalization, the 3-chip camera and 3-dimensional viewing will soon be introduced into clinical practice. Important innovations in the field of instruments are rotating and angulating scissors and dissectors, staplers, and multiclip appliers.

Fig. **172** A special trocar with a blunt tip and a double sealing ring is used in patients with peritoneal adhesions and in the so-called open laparoscopy. The trocar sheath is held in place by means of a spreading mechanism on the abdominal side and sealed off with a rubber sleeve on the outside of the abdomen. The airtight closure thus obtained permits induction and maintenance of the pneumoperitoneum following minilaparotomy

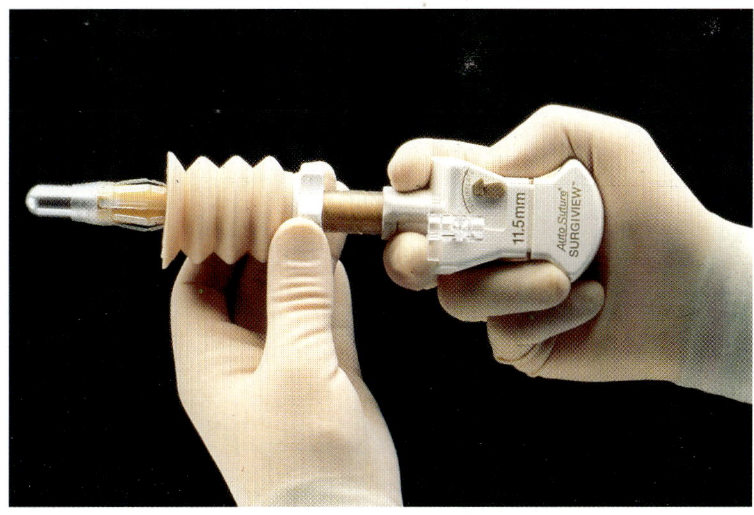

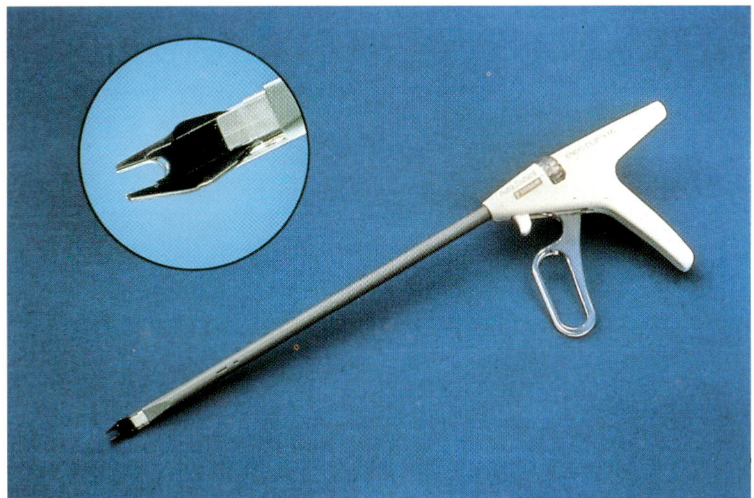

Fig. **173**    The automatically reloading clip applier makes possible repeated use without extraction of the instrument from the abdominal cavity. Titanium clips of various sizes depending on the tissue structures to be secured are available

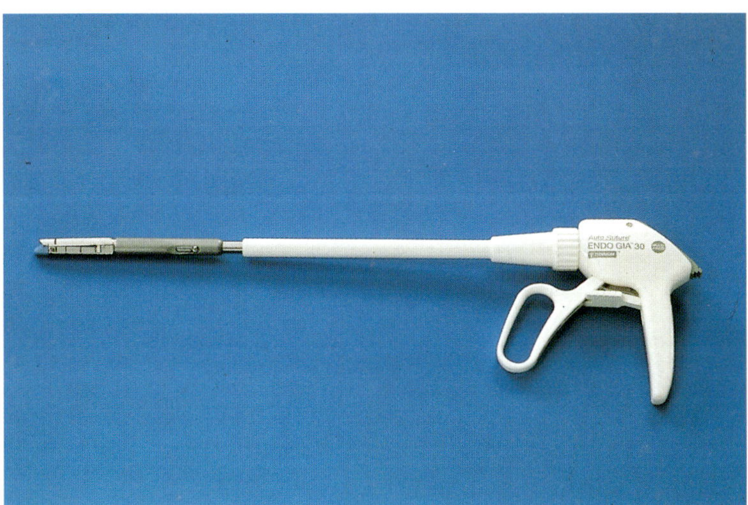

Fig. **174**    The stapler is placed through a 12-mm operating trocar and can be re-loaded repeatedly during a given operation. Blue cartridges with 3.5-mm staples and green cartridges containing staples 4.8 mm long are available. The white cartridge carries the finer vascular staples. Concurrently with the introduction and B-formation of the staples, the tissue is transected between two triple rows of staggered staples

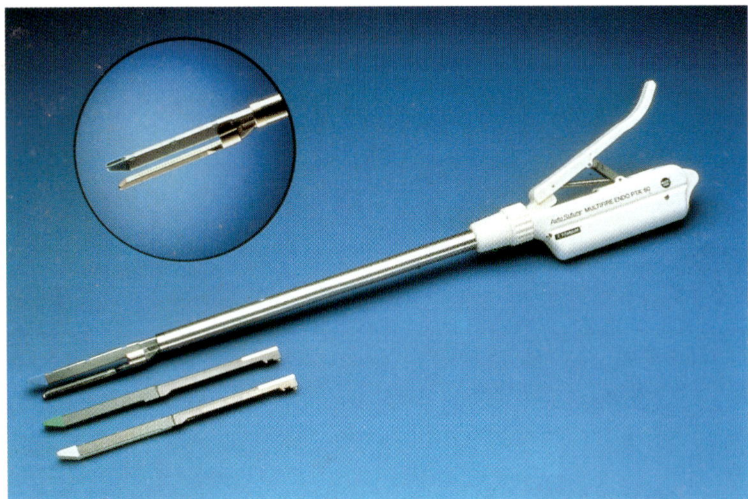

Fig. **175**    With the use of the instrument shown here, tissue structures up to 60 mm in length can be closed on both sides of the simultaneous transection. For thinner tissue the 3.5-mm staples are used, for thicker tissue staples 4.8 mm long are available. The device can be reloaded several times. For the 60-mm instrument, the staple placement and cutting mechanism is activated by compressed air

Fig. **176**   An automatically reloading mechnical suture instrument makes it possible to staple in place or to approximate tissue structures (the peritoneum, for example). Rotation of the head by 320° and angulation by 40° expand the operating range of this instrument

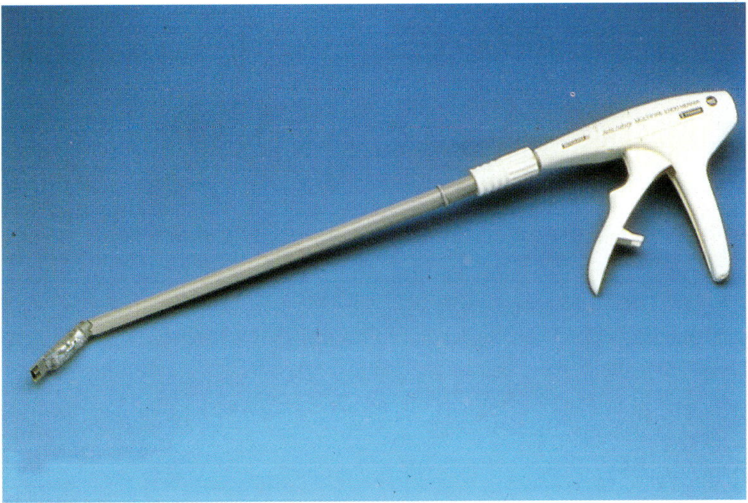

Fig. **177**   The new generation of scissors and dissectors is fitted for the simultaneous use of monopolar thermocautery. The 360° rotation mechanism along the longitudinal axis facilitates dissection

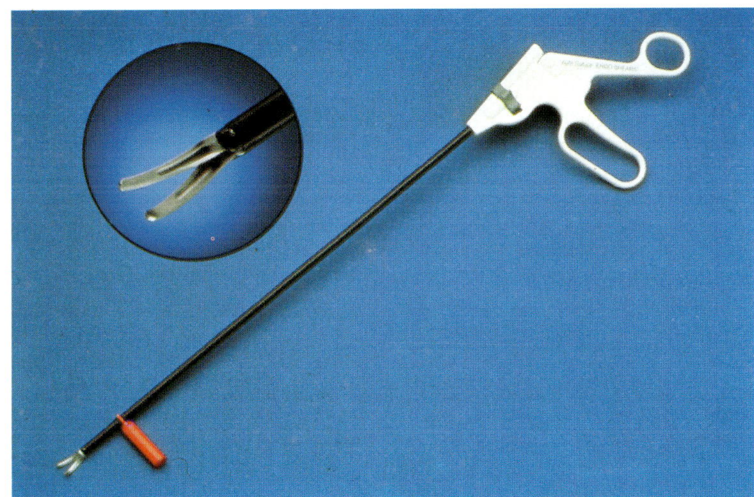

Fig. **178**   Supplementing the rotating instruments, devices that can be angulated by 80° have now become available. This allows the surgeon to expand the operating range of the instruments considerably

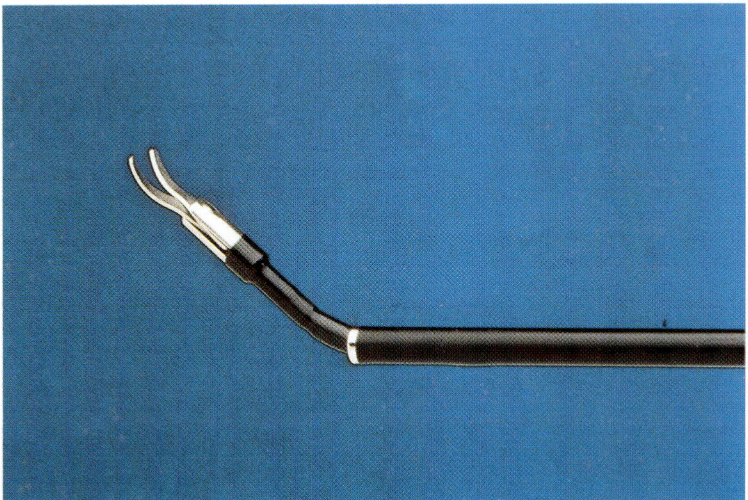

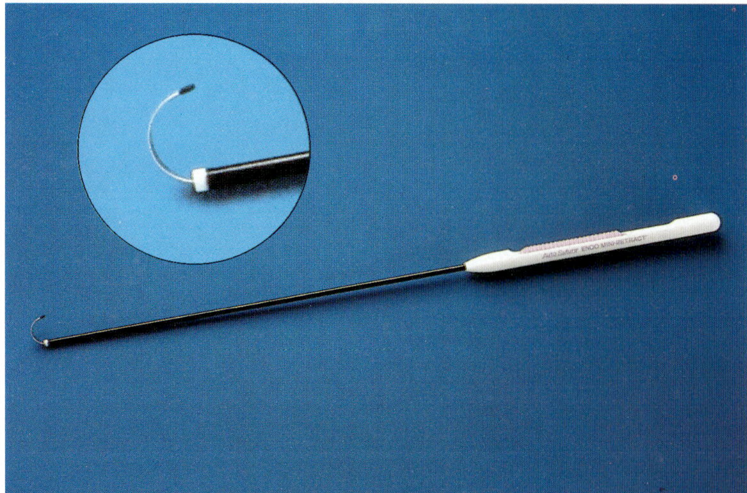

Fig. **179**   The endoretractor with an extensible curved tip is used during dissection, like a probing finger or a Küttner dissector, to free up structures circumferentially

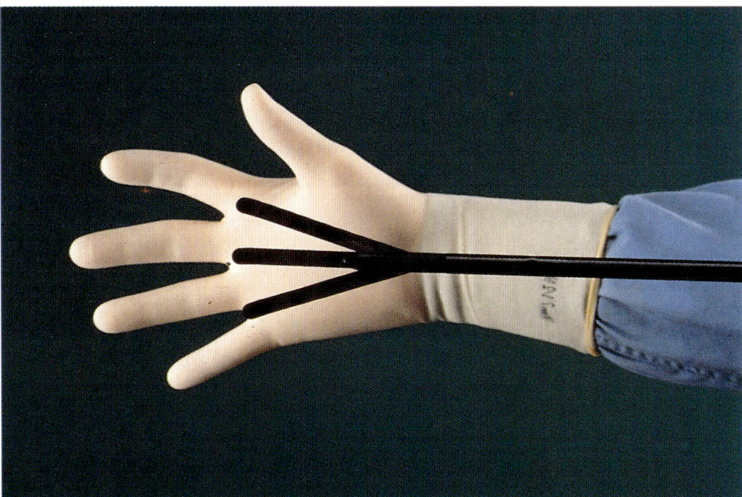

Fig. **180**   After insertion of this retractor into the abdominal cavity, three ribbons can be advanced like a fan, allowing organs to be retracted over a wide area

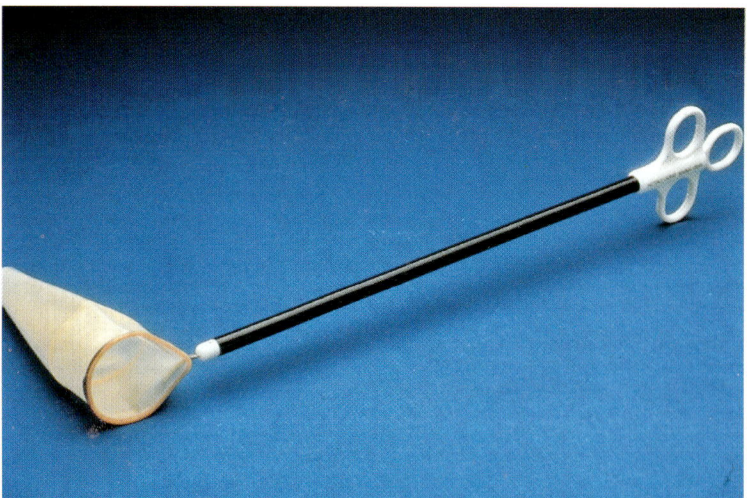

Fig. **181**   Fitted to the tip of the endocatch is a plastic bag which unfolds after insertion into the abdominal cavity. This makes possible the retrieval of lost gallstones or biopsy specimens, for example. The subsequent evacuation eliminates direct contact with the abdominal wall

Fig. **182, 183**  The irrigation–suction unit and its various attachments for the instrument tip such as a pointed, flat, or hooked electrode, has many uses, particularly in the dissection of tissue structures

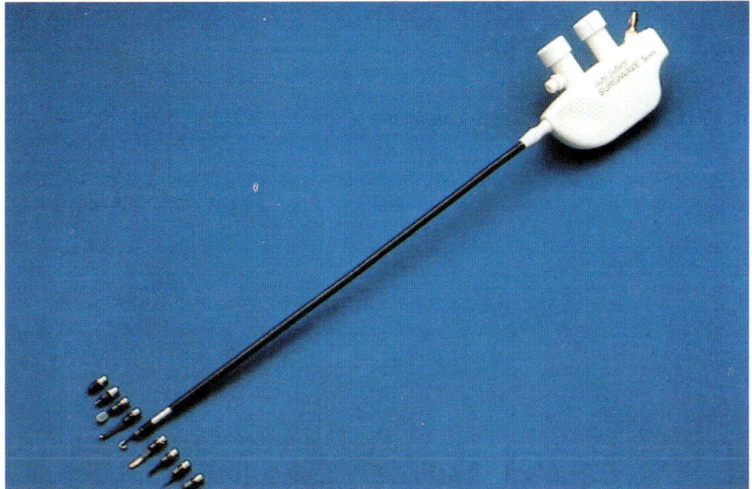

182

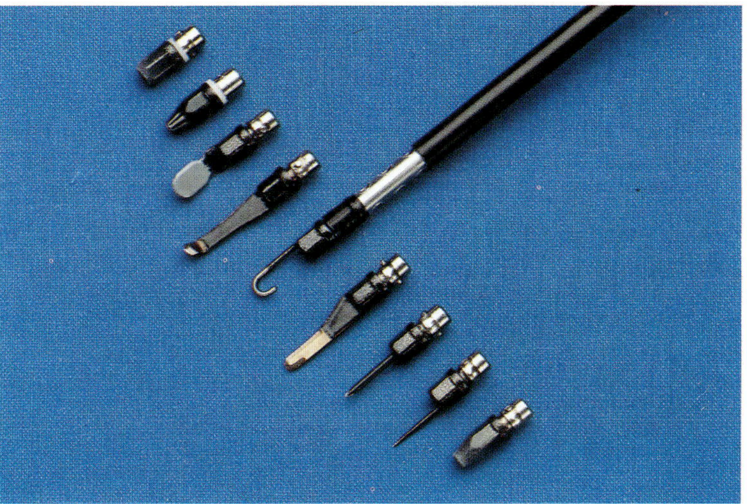

183

# Concluding Remarks and Outlook

Modern laparoscopic techniques have given surgery a timely new dimension, providing for exact anatomical localization and universal accessibility via the video screen and documentation by video film. In addition, surgery is becoming increasingly open to comparison and verification. This is a desirable side-effect, apart from the aforementioned advantages of reduced trauma, better cosmetic results, and shortened hospital stay. Documentation and quality control are accomplished in an almost ideal manner.

The development is exponential at present, with rapidly emerging innovations characterizing this sector of the otherwise tradition-oriented discipline of surgery. A consolidation of confirmed discoveries is not yet at hand; there is a complete lack of controlled studies. Fascination with this exuberance of the novel will spawn new methods. That the indications will be expanded seems likely. In some places, hernias have already been closed from the abdominal side, vagotomies have been performed laparoscopically, cysts have been drained, diverticula have been ablated, and so forth. Which one of these methods will hold its ground, which one represents causal therapy, and which one can stand comparison with conventional procedures remain to be seen in the future. The only certain thing is that fascination with what is technically feasible cannot pass as a justification for its use. With each step, circumspection in weighing the indication and in performing the procedure is of paramount importance. If, for example, in the repair of a hernia only the hernia sac is closed laparoscopically, this cannot take the place of a complete operation. Also, the general anesthesia required is inconsistent with the fact that the extraperitoneal operations for inguinal hernia can be carried out under local anesthesia. In every case, therefore, the dividing line between what is feasible and what is reasonable must not be overlooked.

The obligation to exercise surgical care especially requires the conscientious performance and documentation of laparoscopic operations. In the breaking-in phase, errors are bound to occur; they should be kept to a minimum by training, controls, and self-discipline. The established fact that conventional surgical procedures, such as appendectomy and cholecystectomy, for example, are low-risk standard operations makes it especially incumbent on the laparoscopic surgeon to interpret indications cautiously and to operate with extreme care and technical precision.

Provided these maxims are observed, laparoscopic surgery will soon become part of the regular repertory of modern abdominal surgery.

# References


Barry, R.E., P. Brown, A.E. Read: Physician's use of laporoscopy. Brit. Med. J. 2 (1978) 1276

Berci, G., A. Cuschieri: Practical endoscopy. Baillière Tindall, London 1986

Brantley, J.C., P.M. Riley: Cardiovascular collapse during laparoscopy: a report of two cases. Amer. J. Obstet. Gynecol. 195 (1988) 735

Brown, E.M., V.E. Kunjappan, G.D. Alexander: Fentanyl/alfentanyl for pelvic laparoscopy. Canad. Anaesth. Soc. J. 31 (1984) 251

Brühl, W.: Zwischenfälle und Komplikationen bei der Laparoskopie und gezielten Leberpunktion. Dtsch. med. Wschr. 91 (1966) 2297

Cuschieri, A.: Laparoscopy in general surgery and gastroenterology. Hosp. Med. 24 (1980) 252

Cuschieri, A.: The laparoscopic revolution. J. Roy. Coll. Surgns. Educ. 34 (1990) 295

Cuschieri, A., G. Berci: Laparoscopic biliary surgery. Blackwell, Oxford 1990

Dubois, F., G. Berthelot, H. Levard: Cholécystectomie par coelioscopie. Presse méd. 18 (1989) 980

Fervers, C.: Die Laparoskopie mit dem Zystoskop. Ein Beitrag zur Vereinfachung der Technik und zur endoskopischen Strangdurchtrennung in der Bauchhöhle. Med. Klin. Chir. 178 (1933) 288

Goetze, O.: Ein neues Verfahren der Gasfüllung für das Pneumoperitoneum. Münch. med. Wschr. 51 (1921) 233

Götz, F.: Die endoskopische Appendektomie nach Semm bei den akuten und chronischen Appendizitis. Endosk. heute 2 (1988) 5–7

Götz, F., A. Pier, C. Bacher: Modified laparoscopic appendectomy in surgery. Surg. Endosc. 4 (1990) 6

Hirschowitz, B.I.: Demonstration of a new gastroscope, the "fiber scope". Gastroenterology 35 (1958) 50

Hopkins, H.H.: Optical principles of the endoscope. In: Berci, G.: Endoscopy. Appleton-Century-Crofts, Hemel Hempstead 1976 (p. 3)

Hovorka, J., K. Kortila, O. Erkola: Nitrous oxide does not increase nausea and vomiting following gynecological laparoscopy. Canad. J. Anaesth. 36 (1989) 145

Jakobaeus, H.C.: Über die Möglichkeit, die Zystoskopie bei Untersuchung seröser Höhlen anzuwenden. Münch. med. Wschr. 57 (1910) 2090

Kalk, H., E. Wildhirt: Lehrbuch und Atlas der Laparoskopie und Leberpunktion. Thieme, Stuttgart 1962

Kelling, G.: Oesophagoskopie, Gastroskopie und Zölioskopie. Münch. med. Wschr. 49 (1901) 21

Kenefick, J.P., A. Leader, J.R. Maltoy, P.J. Taylor: Laparoscopy: blood gas values and minor sequelae associated with three techniques based on isoflurane. Brit. J. Anaesth. 59 (1987) 189

Korbsch, R.: Die Laparoskopie nach Jakobaeus. Berl. klin. Wschr. 38 (1921) 696

Kurer, F.L., D.B. Welch: Gynecological laparoscopy: clinical experiences of two anaesthetic techniques. Brit. J. Anaesth. 56 (1984) 1204

Lee, C.M.: Acute hypotension during laparoscopy: a case report Anesth. Analg. 54 (1975) 142

Lindenschmidt, T.-O.: Laparoskopie in der Chirurgie. Therapiewoche 29 (1979) 4096

Motew, M., A.D. Invankovich, J. Bienarz, R.F. Albrecht, B. Zahed, A. Scommegna: Cardiovascular effects and acid-base and blood gas changes during laparoscopy. Amer. J. Obstet. Gynecol. 115 (1973) 1002

Nitze, M.: Eine neue Beleuchtungs- und Untersuchungsmethode für Harnröhre, Harnblase und Rektum. Wien med. Wschr. 24 (1879) 13

Nordentoft, S.: Über Endoskopie geschlossener Cavitäten mittels eines Trokar-Endoskops. Verhandlungen der Dtsch. Ges. für Chirurgie zu Berlin, 1912, 41st Congress. Hirschwald, Berlin 1978

Perrisat, J., D. Collet, R. Belliard: Gallstones: laparoscopic treatment—cholecystectomy, cholecystostomy, and lithotripsy. Our own experiences. Surg. Endosc. 4 (1990) 1

Pier, A., F. Götz, C. Bacher: Laparoscopic app. in 625 cases: from innovation to routine. Surg. Laparosc. Endosc. 1 (1991)

Pier, A., P. Thevissen, B. Ablassmeier: Die Technik der laparoskopischen Cholecystektomie am St. Josef Krankenhaus Linnich—Erfahrungen und Ergebnisse bei 200 Eingriffen. Chirurg 4 (1991)

Reddick, E.J., D.O. Olsen: Laparoscopic laser cholecystectomy. A comparison with mini-lap cholecystectomy. Surg. Endosc. 3 (1989) 131

Riedel, H.H., K. Semm: Das postpelviskopische (laparoskopische) subphrenische Schmerzsyndrom. Arch. Gynäkol. 228 (1979) 283

Roeder, H.: Die Technik der Mandelgesundungsbestrebungen. Ärztl. Rundschau München 57 (1918) 169

Root, B., M.N. Levy, S. Pollack: Gas embolism death after laparoscopy delayed by "trapping" in portal circulation. Anesth. Analg. (Cleveland) 57 (1978) 232

Saleh, J.W.: Peritoneoscopy, an alternative approach to unresolved intra-abdominal disease. Amer. J. Gastroenterol. 6 (1978) 641

Schippers, E., A.P. Öttinger, M. Anuva, M. Polivoda, V. Schumpelick: Intestinale Motilität nach laparoskopischer vs. konventioneller Cholezystektomie: eine tierexperimentelle Studie und klinische Beobachtung. Langenbecks Arch. Chir. 237 (1992) 14–18

Schumpelick, V., E. Schippers: Cholezystektomie – Laparoskopisch oder konventionell. Z. Gastroenterol. (1992)

Semm, K.: Tissue-puncher and loop-ligation. New aids for surgical-therapeutic pelviscopy (laparoscopy) = endoscopic intra-abdominal surgery. Endoscopy 10 (1978) 119

Semm, K.: Statistischer Überblick über die Bauchspiegelung in der Frauenheilkunde bis 1977 in der Bundesrepublik Deutschland. Geburtsh. Frauenheilk. 39 (1979) 537

Semm, K.: Die Automatisierung des Pneumoperitoneums für die endoskopische Abdominalchirugie. Arch. Gynäkol. 232 (1980) 738

Semm, K.: Operationslehre für endoskopische Abdominalchirurgie. Schattauer, Stuttgart 1984

Shandall, A., C. Johnson: Laparoscopy or scanning in oesophageal carcinoma. Brit. J. Surg. 72 (1985) 449

Skacel, M., P. Sengupta, O.M. Plantevin: Morbidity after day case laparoscopy. A comparison of two techniques of tracheal anesthesia. Anesthesia 41 (1986) 537

Stolze, M.: Die Laparoskopie in der chirurgischen Diagnostik. Langenbecks Arch. Chir. 178 (1934) 288

Unverricht, W.: Die Thorakoskopie und Laparoskopie. Berl. Klin. Wschr. 2 (1923) 502

von Ott, D.: Die direkte Beleuchtung der Bauchhöhle, der Harnblase, des Dickdarms und des Uterus zu diagnostischen Zwecken. Rev. Med. Techque. 2 (1909) 27

Wurst, H., U. Finsterer: Pathophysiologische und klinische Aspekte der Laparoskopie. Anästh. Intensivther. Notfallmed. 31 (1990) 187–197

Zimmerman, H.G.: Chirurgische Laparoskopie. Springer, Berlin 1982

# Index